A Global History of Doping in Sport

From turn-of-the-century horseracing to the monolithic anti-doping attitudes now supported by sporting organisations, the development of anti-doping ideology has spread throughout modern sport. Yet heretofore few historians have explored the many ways that international sport has responded to doping. This book seeks to fill that gap by examining different aspects of sport's global efforts to respond to athletes doping. By incorporating cultural, political, and feminist histories that examine international responses to doping, this book aims to better articulate the narrative of doping. The work starts with the first mention of doping in any sport. It examines not only the first efforts to ban doping but also the athletes who sought performance enhancers. Focusing on specific framing events, authors in this book examine the history of doping and how it has indelibly marked the sporting landscape. The result is a work with both breadth and focus. From stories of Japanese swimmers to Italian runners to American jockeys, the work spans the range of doping history. At the same time, the authors remain focused around one single issue: the history of doping in sport.

This book was originally published as a special issue of the *International Journal of the History of Sport.*

John Gleaves is an assistant professor at California State University, Fullerton and the co-director of the International Network of Humanistic Doping Research. His research on doping examines the historical and ethical dimensions of performance-enhancement and the cultural conversation that surrounds the practice. He has authored numerous articles and book chapters exploring the socio-cultural issues related to doping and performance enhancing drugs in sports in refereed journals.

Thomas M. Hunt is an assistant professor of Kinesiology & Health Education at the University of Texas and the H.J. Lutcher Stark Center for Physical Culture and Sports Assistant Director for Academic Affairs. He specialises in the political history of doping in sport as well as sport policy, law, and history. He is the author of many articles on doping and has recently published the book *Drug Games: The International Olympic Committee and the Politics of Doping, 1960–2008*, which examines the history of the International Olympic Committee's reaction to doping.

A Global History of Doping in Sport

Drugs, Policy, and Politics

Edited by
John Gleaves and Thomas M. Hunt

Routledge
Taylor & Francis Group
LONDON AND NEW YORK

First published 2015
by Routledge
2 Park Square, Milton Park, Abingdon, Oxon, OX14 4RN, UK

and by Routledge
711 Third Avenue, New York, NY 10017, USA

Routledge is an imprint of the Taylor & Francis Group, an informa business

British Library Cataloguing in Publication Data
A catalogue record for this book is available from the British Library

ISBN 13: 978-1-138-84094-2

Typeset in Times New Roman
by RefineCatch Limited, Bungay, Suffolk

Publisher's Note
The publisher accepts responsibility for any inconsistencies that may have arisen during the conversion of this book from journal articles to book chapters, namely the possible inclusion of journal terminology.

Disclaimer
Every effort has been made to contact copyright holders for their permission to reprint material in this book. The publishers would be grateful to hear from any copyright holder who is not here acknowledged and will undertake to rectify any errors or omissions in future editions of this book.

Contents

Series Editors' Foreword

On January 1, 2010 *Sport in the Global Society*, created by Professor J. A. Mangan in 1997, was divided into two parts: *Historical Perspectives* and *Contemporary Perspectives*. These new categories involve predominant rather than exclusive emphases. The past is part of the present and the present is part of the past. The Editors of *Historical Perspectives* are Mark Dyreson and Thierry Terret.

The reasons for the division are straightforward. SGS has expanded rapidly since its creation with over one hundred publications in some twelve years. Its editorial teams will now benefit from sectional specialist interests and expertise. *Historical Perspectives* draws on *International Journal of the History of Sport* monograph reviews, themed collections and conference/workshop collections. It is, of course, international in content.

Historical Perspectives continues the tradition established by the original incarnation of *Sport in the Global Society* by promoting the academic study of one of the most significant and dynamic forces in shaping the historical landscapes of human cultures. Sport spans the contemporary globe. It captivates vast audiences. It defines, alters, and reinforces identities for individuals, communities, nations, empires, and the world. Sport organises memories and perceptions, arouses passions and tensions, and reveals harmonies and cleavages. It builds and blurs social boundaries, animating discourses about class, gender, race, and ethnicity. Sport opens new vistas on the history of human cultures, intersecting with politics and economics, ideologies and theologies. It reveals aesthetic tastes and energises consumer markets.

By the end of the twentieth century a critical mass of scholars recognised the importance of sport in their analyses of human experiences and *Sport in the Global Society* emerged to provide an international outlet for the world's leading investigators of the subject. As Professor Mangan contended in the original series foreword: 'The story of modern sport is the story of the modern world – in microcosm; a modern global tapestry permanently being woven. Furthermore, nationalist and imperialist, philosopher and politician, radical and conservative have all sought in sport a manifestation of national identity, status and superiority. Finally for countless millions sport is the personal pursuit of ambition, assertion, well-being and enjoyment.'

Sport in the Global Society: Historical Perspectives continues the project, building on previous work in the series and excavating new terrain. It remains a consistent and coherent response to the attention the academic community demands for the serious study of sport.

Mark Dyreson
Thierry Terret

SPORT IN THE GLOBAL SOCIETY –
HISTORICAL PERSPECTIVES

Series Editors: Mark Dyreson and Thierry Terret

A GLOBAL HISTORY OF
DOPING IN SPORT

Sport in the Global Society: Historical Perspectives
Series Editors: Mark Dyreson and Thierry Terret

As Robert Hands in *The Times* recently observed, the growth of sports studies in recent years has been considerable. This unique series with over one hundred volumes in the last decade has played its part. Politically, culturally, emotionally and aesthetically, sport is a major force in the modern world. Its impact will grow as the world embraces ever more tightly the contemporary secular trinity: the English language, technology and sport. *Sport in the Global Society* will continue to record sport's phenomenal progress across the world stage.

Titles in the Series

A Global History of Doping in Sport
Drugs, Policy, and Politics
Edited by John Gleaves and Thomas Hunt

American National Pastimes – A History
Edited by Mark Dyreson and Jaime Schultz

Delivering Olympic and Elite Sport in a Cross Cultural Context
From Beijing to London
Edited by Fan Hong and Lu Zhouxiang

East Asia, Geopolitics and the 2012 London Games
Edited by J. A. Mangan and Marcus Chu

Encoding the Olympics
The Beijing Olympic Games and the Communication Impact Worldwide
Edited by Luo Qing and Giuseppe Richeri

Gymnastics, a Transatlantic Movement
From Europe to America
Edited by Gertrud Pfister

London, Europe and the Olympic Games
Historical Perspectives
Edited by Thierry Terret

'Manufactured' Masculinity
Making Imperial Manliness, Morality and Militarism
J. A. Mangan

Mapping an Empire of American Sport
Expansion, Assimilation, Adaptation
Edited by Mark Dyreson, J. A. Mangan and Roberta J. Park

Militarism, Hunting, Imperialism
'Blooding' The Martial Male
J. A. Mangan and Callum McKenzie

Olympic Aspirations
Realised and Unrealised
Edited by J. A. Mangan and Mark Dyreson

Post-Beijing 2008: Geopolitics, Sport and the Pacific Rim
Edited by J. A. Mangan and Fan Hong

Representing the Nation
Sport and Spectacle in Post-Revolutionary Mexico
Claire and Keith Brewster

Rule Britannia: Nationalism, Identity and the Modern Olympic Games
Matthew Llewellyn

Soft Power Politics – Football and Baseball in the Western Pacific Rim
Edited by Rob Hess, Peter Horton and J. A. Mangan

Sport and Emancipation of European Women
The Struggle for Self-fulfilment
Edited by Gigliola Gori and J. A. Mangan

Sport and Nationalism in Asia
Power, Politics and Identity
Edited by Fan Hong and Lu Zhouxiang

Sport, Bodily Culture and Classical Antiquity in Modern Greece
Edited by Eleni Fournaraki and Zinon Papakonstantinou

Sport in the Cultures of the Ancient World
New Perspectives
Edited by Zinon Papakonstantinou

Sport in the Middle East
Edited by Fan Hong

Sport in the Pacific
Colonial and Postcolonial Consequencies
Edited by C. Richard King

Sport, Literature, Society
Cultural Historical Studies
Edited by Alexis Tadié, J. A. Mangan and Supriya Chaudhuri

Sport, Militarism and the Great War
Martial Manliness and Armageddon
Edited by Thierry Terret and J. A. Mangan

Sport Past and Present in South Africa
(Trans)forming the Nation
Edited by Scarlet Cornelissen and Albert Grundlingh

The Asian Games: Modern Metaphor for 'The Middle Kingdom' Reborn
Political Statement, Cultural Assertion, Social Symbol
Edited by J. A. Mangan, Marcus P. Chu and Dong Jinxia

The Balkan Games and Balkan Politics in the Interwar Years 1929–1939
Politicians in Pursuit of Peace
Penelope Kissoudi

The Beijing Olympics: Promoting China
Soft and Hard Power in Global Politics
Edited by Kevin Caffrey

The History of Motor Sport
A Case Study Analysis
Edited by David Hassan

The New Geopolitics of Sport in East Asia
Edited by William Kelly and J. A. Mangan

The Politicisation of Sport in Modern China
Communists and Champions
Fan Hong and Lu Zhouxiang

The Politics of the Male Body in Sport
The Danish Involvement
Hans Bonde

The Rise of Stadiums in the Modern United States
Cathedrals of Sport
Edited by Mark Dyreson and Robert Trumpbour

The Triple Asian Olympics
Asia Rising – the Pursuit of National Identity, International Recognition and Global Esteem
Edited by J. A. Mangan, Sandra Collins and Gwang Ok

The Triple Asian Olympics – Asia Ascendant
Media, Politics and Geopolitics
Edited by J. A. Mangan, Luo Qing and Sandra Collins

The Visual in Sport
Edited by Mike Huggins and Mike O'Mahony

Women, Sport, Society
Further Reflections, Reaffirming Mary Wollstonecraft
Edited by Roberta Park and Patricia Vertinsky

Citation Information

The chapters in this book were originally published in the *International Journal of the History of Sport*, volume 31, issue 8 (April 2014). When citing this material, please use the original page numbering for each article, as follows:

Chapter 1
Introduction: A Global History of Doping in Sport: Drugs, Nationalism and Politics
John Gleaves
International Journal of the History of Sport, volume 31, issue 8 (April 2014) pp. 815–819

Chapter 2
Pierre de Coubertin, Doped 'Amateurs' and the 'Spirit of Sport': The Role of Mythology in Olympic Anti-Doping Policies
Ian Ritchie
International Journal of the History of Sport, volume 31, issue 8 (April 2014) pp. 820–838

Chapter 3
Sport, Drugs and Amateurism: Tracing the Real Cultural Origins of Anti-Doping Rules in International Sport
John Gleaves and Matthew Llewellyn
International Journal of the History of Sport, volume 31, issue 8 (April 2014) pp. 839–853

Chapter 4
A Powerful False Positive: Nationalism, Science and Public Opinion in the 'Oxygen Doping' Allegations Against Japanese Swimmers at the 1932 Olympics
Mark Dyreson and Thomas Rorke
International Journal of the History of Sport, volume 31, issue 8 (April 2014) pp. 854–870

Chapter 5
The Myth of the Nazi Steroid
Marcel Reinold and John Hoberman
International Journal of the History of Sport, volume 31, issue 8 (April 2014) pp. 871–883

Chapter 6

The Emergence of Moral Technopreneurialism in Sport: Techniques in Anti-Doping Regulation, 1966–1976
Kathryn Henne
International Journal of the History of Sport, volume 31, issue 8 (April 2014) pp. 884–901

Chapter 7

Drugs, the Law, and the Downfall of Dancer's Image at the 1968 Kentucky Derby: A Case Study on Human Conceptions of Domesticated Animals
Thomas M. Hunt, Scott R. Jedlicka and Matthew T. Bowers
International Journal of the History of Sport, volume 31, issue 8 (April 2014) pp. 902–913

Chapter 8

Minor Problems: The Recognition of Young Athletes in the Development of International Anti-Doping Policies
Sarah Teetzel and Marcus Mazzucco
International Journal of the History of Sport, volume 31, issue 8 (April 2014) pp. 914–933

Chapter 9

Who Guards the Guardians?
Verner Møller
International Journal of the History of Sport, volume 31, issue 8 (April 2014) pp. 934–950

Chapter 10

Why Lance Armstrong? Historical Context and Key Turning Points in the 'Cleaning Up' of Professional Cycling
Paul Dimeo
International Journal of the History of Sport, volume 31, issue 8 (April 2014) pp. 951–968

Please direct any queries you may have about the citations to
clsuk.permissions@cengage.com

INTRODUCTION

A Global History of Doping in Sport: Drugs, Nationalism and Politics

John Gleaves

California State University, Fullerton

The philosopher Ludwig Wittgenstein admonished his fellow philosophers, saying 'Don't think, but look!'[1] Wittgenstein protested his field's desire to overly theoritise in lieu of actually going out into the messy world and getting some mud on their boots. It is not that thinking, or theory, was bad – after all, Wittgenstein was a philosopher – but it is that the thinking, when it replaces looking, when it comes before looking, can cause investigations to miss the very phenomena they are after. We mistake our assumptions and theories for immutable truths and miss the inconvenient messiness that often lurks in the real world. To grasp the important things, Wittgenstein concluded, we need not do more reasoning or theoretising, but rather look more attentively at what lies before us.

Such an admonition from the likes of Wittgenstein seemed appropriate for the historical understanding of doping research. From Lance Armstrong and Barry Bonds to the Cold War 'Big Arms' race between the USA and the Soviet Union and rumours of Nazi steroid use, sport and stories about performance-enhancing substances capture the public imagination.[2] This interest has generated numerous discussions among academics as well as the media and the general public, who in large part reference historical examples to illustrate general lessons about the nature of doping. Yet such conversations – as well as some academic writing – have come littered with myths, half-truths and unverified assumptions.[3] However, recent work has illustrated the value of the 'Don't think, but look' approach and deconstructed a handful of these historical narratives, questioning their accuracy and functional value and illustrating the ability for historians to shed insights on culturally loaded topics.[4]

Why is Wittgenstein's quote to 'Don't think, but look' so prescient for the field of sport history in general and doping in particular? The historian Paul Dimeo self-reflexively notes in the prologue to his work *A History of Drug Use in Sport* that he

> had been reading around in sports history, thinking of getting into the methodological debates then emerging on textuality, discourse and representation. The question of doping and anti-doping seemed ripe for a deconstructionist-type approach that unpicked the cultural and political values underpinning the ostensibly 'good' anti-doping ideology ... However, it was frustrating to read, in so many different places, passages of historical narrative that failed to meet even the most fundamental requirements of reasonably good historiography. They did not use primary sources, they unquestioningly repeated secondary sources that contained no evidence, they used invented stories from the past to prove points about the present, and they failed to ask any contextual questions.[5]

Dimeo's frustration grew in the case of Arthur Linton, a Welsh cyclist widely cited as the first ever death from doping. Citations for Linton's death range from academic publications by Barrie Houlihan and Ivan Waddington to institutional claims found on the website of the World Anti-Doping Agency and the United Nation's UNESCO report on drugs in sport.[6] The claim, more or less, holds that Arthur Linton died after the Bordeaux–Paris race of 1886 after taking trimethyl. How these authors arrived at such hard evidence is unclear since the authors provide no citations of any record or any good source of evidence. Reproducing uncited claims is bad enough, but even worse, Dimeo points out, is that this story is a falsehood. Based on contemporary media accounts including his obituary in the *London Times*, we can say that Linton did not die in 1886 but in 1896, not from drugs but from typhoid fever, and successfully won more cycling races in the decade between his alleged death and his obituary's publication. Such evidence should at least cast doubt for any scholar wishing to cite Linton's death as the earliest example of a doping-related fatality.[7]

Now to be sure, there are objective historical facts. History cannot be written any which way. And while how historians interpret and understand these facts is a subjective process laden with biases and reflexivity and the sources historians use do not exist inert in a valueless state, it is also true that historians can, more or less, get closer to these objective facts by looking. It also seems useful for these more or less verified facts to guide historical analysis and context; with such facts in place, historians can begin making sense of the past in ways that mean something to the present.

This process, which each author has contributed to, is so important in historical scholarship because, as Dimeo noted, the field of doping is ripe with myths and unquestioned stories. A case in point was that of the Danish cyclist Knud Enemark Jensen. Jensen, the first athlete to ever die during an Olympic Games, was alleged to have died from amphetamines at the 1960 Rome Olympic Games. News reports went so far as to allege the amphetamines as the cause of death and you can still find today sources linking the stimulants to Jensen's demise. However, like Linton, this story turned out not to be true. The Danish scholar Verner Møller examined the case and found no evidence of Jensen's use of amphetamines. Møller, citing the direct language from the autopsy report, concluded that 'the death of Knud Enemark Jensen was caused solely by heatstroke' and that post-mortem examinations showed no signs of amphetamines.[8] True, Jensen had taken a vasodiollator roniacol (the opposite of a stimulant) which may have worsened his condition, but this still does not support the press accounts linking his death to amphetamines. In fact, on the World Anti-Doping Agency's website, you can still find the following: 'The death of Danish cyclist Knud Enemark Jensen during competition at the Olympic Games in Rome 1960 (the autopsy revealed traces of amphetamine) increased the pressure for sports authorities to introduce drug testing'.[9] So I point this story out as simply a tale of caution. We must critically consider our sources and, when citing documents which we have not accessed, must be sure to note this fact.

As mentioned previously, the historiography of doping illustrates a proclivity towards accepting certain truths – that doping causes death, was not banned until after a cyclist died or contradicts the tradition of sport – that conform with popular views of doping today. This, as the behavioural psychologist Daniel Kahneman argued, is a common cognitive fallacy known as confirmation bias.[10] Confirmation bias is the tendency to interpret information in a way that confirms one's preconceptions. In academia, where scholars tend to reproduce accepted views through citations and references to secondary work, confirmation bias becomes even easier so that when Waddington cited Houlihan's recounting of Linton's death, preconceptions become strengthened into accepted paradigms. With Jensen's death, the willingness to believe a cyclist died from amphetamines, despite no evidence supporting this claim, still lives on in popular lore.

To protect against such bias, scholars would do well to go back and look at original documents and sources whenever possible. Archives, rule books, visual and material sources, and even, when possible, oral histories can challenge assumptions by providing some checks to either, as our authors showed, confirm or contradict the myths that exist in popular culture. That is not to say that these sources somehow count as the 'truth' and historians must reconstruct these sources into one narrative that captures what the past was really like. But they can provide evidence to inform historians as they pursue a more accurate understanding of the past.

Let me provide one personal example. While at the Brundage archives in Champaign, Illinois, I was flipping through a file on amateurism when out fell a yellowed piece of notebook paper. Scribbled in Avery Brundage's own handwriting, I realised the hasty drafting of the IOC's first anti-doping statement from 1937. Excited, I jumped back, banging my elbow and knocking my chair to the ground, completely disrupting all of the other scholars working silently in the archive. But this piece of paper led to the examination of the IOC's decision to ratify nine amendments to the IOC's amateurism rule, Rule 26. But my colleague, Matthew Llewellyn, and I assumed these amendments, passed on the verge of World War II, were forgotten, and we thought we had a great story of a 'forgotten reform'. We scanned the popular presses in English, German and French – sources likely to cover IOC reforms – and found no coverage of the IOC's decision to ban doping, further confirming the event simply had been forgotten as Tokyo's bid fell apart and Europe drifted towards war. More importantly, we assumed it was forgotten because prevalent historiography, including the works of Paul Dimeo, Verner Møller and many others, dates the IOC ban on doping to the years following Jensen's death at the 1960 Rome Games.[11] But when we went to check the 1946 Charter, the first charter published following the IOC's amendments in 1938, we found the exact amendments published under Rule 26.[12] But surely they were dropped sometime between 1946 and 1960, we thought. How else could such scholars have made the claim that no rule prohibited doping at the time of Jensen's death? But when we checked the subsequent Olympic Charters, including and past Jensen's death, sure enough the same language handwritten by Brundage, with only slight modifications over the years, had existed in every charter since 1946.

The point is the need for historians to go look, especially when it comes to the issue of doping. As authors in this collection illustrate, the issues that surrounded the doping look very different than how they are often portrayed today. Ian Ritchie illustrates how the role of mythology and ideas about chivalry shaped Pierre de Coubertin's notions of amateurism and doping. Mathew Llewellyn and I examined the cultural origins of anti-doping attitudes and how they entered into the Olympic Movement. Mark Dyreson and Thomas Rorke capture a 'tempest in a teapot', which shows how nationalism and public pride can drive accusations of doping and dubious conduct, while Marcel Reinold and John Hoberman deconstruct the long-held myth linking the Nazi athletes to steroids. Introducing the term 'Technoprenuralism', Kathryn Henne traces the rise of an industry built upon enforcing anti-doping rules. On the other side, Thomas Hunt, Scott Jedlicka and Matthew Bowers wade through legal briefs and they identify how a case involving doping and horse racing played to anthropomorphised ideals, while Sarah Teetzel and Marcus Mazzucco examine the underexplored world of minors and international doping policy. Turning towards more recent issues, Verner Møller examines the increasing autonomy and power of those charged with guarding sports' moral interest, and Paul Dimeo examines cycling's efforts to rid itself of doping through the case of Lance Armstrong.

These authors showed that the history of doping needs to be reconsidered because the changes in our own society's views on the subject may obscure how past generations understood the issue. More importantly, the styles of social thought that we take for granted about doping were not the same as those in the past. This can lead to a misreading or an inventing of history that reinterprets past stories to fit the needs of the present. Such insights illustrate why history and ethnography demand constant rewriting. Returning to these events is valuable when historians gain new evidence, like unexamined archival stories or when popular lore has led to the misreading of past events. But more importantly, as the questions historians and ethnographers ask change, like in the case of doping where popular social beliefs strongly condemn such practices, the 'don't think but look' approach can help us as we investigate how past doping issues unfolded and how they influence present doping attitudes. In this sense, we do well to remind ourselves of Wittgenstein's appeal and take the time to look for ourselves.

Acknowledgements

Thomas Hunt and I wish to thank the many anonymous reviewers whose valued time and valuable insights significantly improved the final product. We are grateful for their unsung efforts.

Notes

1. Wittgenstein, *Philosophical Investigations*, 66.
2. Examples of literature that cover these issues include Dimeo, *History of Drug Use in Sport*; Hoberman, *Mortal Engines* and Hunt, *Drug Games.*
3. An example is Goldman, *Death in the Locker Room.*
4. For example, see López, "Invention of a 'Drug of Mass Destruction'," 84–109; Møller, "Knud Enemark Jensen's Death During the 1960 Rome Olympics," 452–71.
5. Dimeo, *History of Drug Use in Sport,* x.
6. Houlihan, *Dying to Win*; Waddington, *Sport, Health and Drugs*; "A Brief History of Anti-Doping" (*World Anti-Doping Agency*, accessed April 11, 2014, http://www.wada-ama.org/en/about-wada/history/a-brief-history-of-anti-doping/) and "International Convention Against Doping in Sport" (*UNESCO*, accessed April 11, 2014, http://www.unesco.org/new/en/social-and-human-sciences/themes/anti-doping/international-convention-against-doping-in-sport/).
7. Dimeo, *History of Drug Use in Sport*, 7–8.
8. Møller, "Knud Enemark Jensen's Death During the 1960 Rome Olympics," 469.
9. "A Brief History of Anti-Doping" (*World Anti-Doping Agency*, accessed April 11, 2014, http://www.wada-ama.org/en/about-wada/history/a-brief-history-of-anti-doping/).
10. Kahneman, *Thinking Fast and Slow.*
11. Dimeo, *History of Drug Use in Sport*, 103; Hunt, *Drug Games*, ix; Møller, "Knud Enemark Jensen's Death During the 1960 Rome Olympics," 465 and Waddington and Smith, *Introduction to Drugs in Sport*, 8 and 18.
12. International Olympic Committee, "Olympic Rules, 1946," 28.

References

Dimeo, P. *A History of Drug Use in Sport 1876–1976: Beyond Good and Evil.* New York: Routledge, 2007.

Goldman, B. *Death in the Locker Room: Steroids, Cocaine & Sports.* Tucson, AZ: Body Press, 1984.

Hoberman, J. *Mortal Engines: The Science of Performance and the Dehumanization of Sport.* New York: Free Press, 1992.

Houlihan, B. *Dying to Win: Doping in Sport and the Development of Anti-Doping Policy.*, 2nd ed. Strasbourg: Council of Europe, 2002.

Hunt, T. *Drug Games: The International Olympic Committee and the Politics of Doping, 1960–2008.* Austin: University of Texas Press, 2011.

International Olympic Committee. "Olympic Rules, 1946." Accessed April 11, 2014. p. 28. http://www.olympic.org/Documents/Olympic%20Charter/Olympic_Charter_through_time/1946-Olympic_Charter.pdf

Kahneman, D. *Thinking, Fast and Slow.* New York: Farrar, Straus and Giroux, 2011.

López, Bernat. "The Invention of a 'Drug of Mass Destruction': Deconstructing the EPO Myth." *Sport in History* 31, no. 1 (2011): 84–109.
Møller, V. "Knud Enemark Jensen's Death During the 1960 Rome Olympics: A Search for Truth?" *Sport in History* 25, no. 3 (2005): 452–471.
Waddington, Ivan. *Sport, Health and Drugs: A Critical Sociological Perspective.* New York: E & FN Spon, 2000.
Waddington, Ivan, and Andy Smith. *An Introduction to Drugs in Sport: Addicted to Winning?* New York: Routledge, 2009.
Wittgenstein, Ludwig. *Philosophical Investigations.*, 3rd Ed. Oxford: Basil Blackwell, 1996.

Pierre de Coubertin, Doped 'Amateurs' and the 'Spirit of Sport': The Role of Mythology in Olympic Anti-Doping Policies

Ian Ritchie

Department of Kinesiology, Brock University, Canada

The central justification for the prohibition of drugs in the Olympic Games is that drugs are contrary to the 'spirit of sport'. This paper considers the 'spirit of sport' claim by placing Olympic ideals in their full, historical relief. The central thesis is that the recent prohibition against performance-enhancing substances based on the ideal of the 'spirit of sport' is in fact part of a much longer historical project to proffer an image of the Olympics as a 'pure' form of sport. The ideals and 'foundation myths' of Olympic founder Pierre de Coubertin are first used as a comparative point upon which to study major changes to Olympic sport in the twentieth century and the construction of anti-doping policies. Coubertin built his system of myths around sport from three epochs: ancient, medieval and modern. The study then moves on to consider two important historical periods in the Olympic movement: the first three decades of the twentieth century and the period from just after WWII to the early 1970s. During both time periods, major challenges to Coubertin's original foundation myths are considered alongside attempts on the part of the International Olympic Committee to sanction performance-enhancing substances and methods. The foundation myths upon which Coubertin built his movement are also essential elements of anti-doping regulations.

Introduction

What, exactly, is the 'spirit of sport'? At the most obvious level, in terms of anti-doping policy the World Anti-Doping Agency's *World Anti-Doping Code* justifies the ban on certain substances and methods based on the premise that they contradict sport's spirit: 'Anti-doping programs seek to preserve what is intrinsically valuable about sport' the *Code* states as its 'Fundamental Rationale'. 'This intrinsic value is often referred to as "the spirit of sport", it is the essence of Olympism.' The *Code* also goes on to list a host of sub-values that characterise sport's spirit, including 'fair play', 'health', 'excellence', 'character and education' and 'joy'.[1]

The 'spirit of sport' language has become prominent since the creation of the World Anti-Doping Agency's first *Code* in 2003. However, the Olympic Games has always proffered images of 'timelessness' of itself as an event and 'purity' of its brand of sport; the same was true in Pierre de Coubertin's time as it is today.[2] The *Code's* reference to Olympic 'essence' is in truth a continuation of a long tradition. Writing in *Fortnightly Review* in 1908, Coubertin described his newly founded event as 'something else' and 'not to be found in any other variety of athletic competition'. Counter-posing his Games to the 'dangerous canker' of 'unbridled competition' that was emerging in the increasingly professionalised and commercialised world of sport in the late nineteenth and early twentieth centuries, Coubertin claimed that the model of ancient Greek sport would act as a 'regulator' to preserve the 'Spirit of fair play' in his Olympic movement. After all, it was at Olympia, Coubertin claimed, that 'athleticism ... remained pure and magnificent'.[3]

It is now well known that Coubertin's account of the ancient Games was premised on a combination of mythology, based on the knowledge and sources available to him during the late nineteenth century, alongside his own political objectives in convincing others that reinstating 'his' Olympic movement was a worthwhile endeavour.[4] Irrespective of the many false notions that Coubertin gleaned from his reading and interpretation of ancient Greece, his ability to link the nascent modern movement to ancient times was, as Bruce Kidd points out, 'a genius stroke of public relations' because the image of a sport movement based on an everlasting 'essential' element of the human condition helped Coubertin overcome the struggles of competing groups over the ultimate purpose of sport while simultaneously drawing attention away from the restricted class traditions upon which the Games were founded.[5] It gave Coubertin's movement, in other words, 'rightful ownership' of sport and this helped set the foundation for the claim of 'purity' and 'permanence' in the decades to come.

The central argument of this study is that the current underlying 'philosophical' foundation for anti-doping regulations is in fact a continuation of the 'foundation myths' in the Olympic movement created by Coubertin in the late nineteenth century.[6] Despite dramatic changes to 'sport' in the twentieth century, the Olympic Games always maintained and perpetuated a 'purity' of sport myth. The manner in which that myth has been perpetuated has changed, as we shall see. However, while Olympic mythology's storyline has changed, the overriding script has always been the same – Olympic sport's 'purity' and the Games as 'an event' have always been two major components of the movement's mythological system.

The analysis focuses on the original foundation myths of Coubertin and their importance in the early stages of the Games. Myths based on references to ancient, modern and, in particular, medieval sport are highlighted. The various challenges to those foundation myths in the early stages of the Games – roughly, from 1896 to the 1930s – and, subsequently, the post-WWII period leading up to the dissolution of the amateur clause in the Olympic Charter in the early 1970s are traced. In both cases, the manner in which Coubertin's foundation myths both were perpetuated and challenged is discussed. Also, in both periods, the challenge 'doping' made to Olympic authorities, and the manner in which foundation myths were utilised to create anti-doping policies, is described. Because of the extensive time periods covered in this study alongside the diverse topics discussed, an eclectic range of sources is used – primary references are used whenever possible, in particular in discussing Coubertin's ideas or Olympic policies regarding anti-doping or amateurism, alongside several secondary sources.

Foundations of 'Purity' in the Early Modern Games

The 'foundation myths' that Coubertin built were important for two reasons. First, we should always remember that his ideals for the Games were not myths for Coubertin. They were based on his extensive reading of literature, philosophy, politics, education, history and several other areas, and they were based on well-respected sources available to him in his day. Second, and perhaps more importantly, the images of grandeur, universalism and purity he created for 'his' social movement were significant because they played a crucial role in overcoming the real-world financial, organisational and political obstacles that he faced in the nascent days of the movement. In short, Coubertin could not achieve his goal of building the Games as a social movement aimed towards pedagogical reform, overcome the varied political agendas of various sports administrators in different nations in Europe and elsewhere, nor was he able to prevent Greece from surpassing his goals in favour of its own nationalistic interests leading up to the inaugural Games in 1896 without shaping in peoples' minds a sense that his movement represented a universal version of sport that had essentialist characteristics and was 'pure'.[7]

Sophisticated in propaganda and social marketing, Coubertin took full advantage of image-creating techniques to garner support for his fledging movement.[8] Early in 1894 when Coubertin sent out his invitation to the 'International Congress of Amateurs' to be held at Paris's Sorbonne University in the summer of that year, he knew that, first, holding the event at such a prestigious location in-and-of-itself had considerable cachet. On the opening day of the conference, invited delegates sat in the Sorbonne's grand amphitheatre where they listened to speeches, drank Champaign, listened to an ode to athleticism by well-known French poet Jean Aicard and soaked in a musical performance of the 'Delphic Hymn to Apollo' based on inscribed tablets discovered at Delphi only one year earlier, all the while surrounded by the famous French painter Pierre Puvis de Chavannes's neo-classical mural *Le Bois sacré* [The Sacred Wood].[9] 'It seemed to me', Coubertin later claimed, 'that under the venerable roof of the Sorbonne the words "Olympic Games" would resound more impressively and persuasively on the audience'.[10] Citing the effect of the Delphic Hymn in particular as 'immense', Coubertin's wish to have his modern sports movement linked to ancient Greece could not have been more fully realised: 'Hellenism thus infiltrated the vast enclosure. In these first hours, the Congress had come to a head. Henceforth I knew ... no one would vote against the restoration of the Olympic Games.'[11]

Second, the conference itself was in some respects a ruse for Coubertin to achieve his lofty aspirations for the revival of the Games. Knowing that support for the revival of an 'Olympic Games' was mixed at best, Coubertin enticed defenders of amateurism – what David Young refers to, likely without too much historical exaggeration, as 'the fetish of the aristocrats' – from around the world with a misleading title 'International Congress of Amateurs' and a preliminary eight-item programme that emphasised the conditions of amateur rules in the first seven items but the possibility of reviving an Olympic Games inauspiciously as the eighth.[12] However, upon their arrival, Coubertin's true intentions were made plain to the delegates; the title of the Congress's programme read that the gathering's purpose was 'For the Reestablishment of the Olympic Games'.[13] Young demonstrates quite clearly that Coubertin's ruse was entirely deliberate; he admitted later in his life that amateurism was a 'screen' and that his interest in amateurism leading up to the conference was 'zeal without real conviction'.[14] However, the first major paragraph in the original circulation sent to potential delegates in January of 1894 in fact gave clues to Coubertin's ultimate objectives. Indeed, this paragraph is worth quoting at length because within these words we see Coubertin's realisation that he needed to cater to the needs of amateur 'fetishes' of the day alongside the underlying philosophical and historical foundation upon which Coubertin wanted the Games to be built:

> First and foremost, it is vital that athletics retain the noble and chivalrous quality which distinguished it in the past, so that it can effectively continue to play within the education of modern peoples the admirable role which the Greek masters attributed to it. Human imperfection tends always to transform the Olympian athlete into a circus gladiator. One must

> choose between two athletic methods which are not compatible. To defend oneself against the spirit of lucre and professionalism which threatens to invade them, the Amateurs, in the majority of countries, have created complicated legislation full of compromises and contradictions; what is more, too often the letter rather than the spirit of this legislation is respected.[15]

What, for Coubertin, inspired the true 'spirit' of the otherwise overly 'complicated' legislation of amateurism? The underlying 'spirit' of Olympism, as is now well known from historical accounts, lay not in amateurism *per se*, but in much deeper ideals based on conservative ideas prevalent in his day.

Rob Beamish points out that Coubertin was heavily influenced by the conservative tradition in Europe in the nineteenth century. The writings of Joseph de Maistre, Louis de Bonald, Hugues Felicité de Lamnennais and René de Chateaubriand in France and Edmund Burke in England were all important. The conservative tradition emphasised several interrelated ideals, including the privileging of the social whole over individual rights and the biological analogy of interrelated functioning parts leading to the smooth functioning of the whole – 'A Society Is an Organism' as Herbert Spencer stated bluntly in his *Principles of Sociology* in 1898.[16] The tradition also believed in the integrating force of religion, in particular Roman Catholicism, alongside its adherence to the 'great chain of being' and the natural, hierarchical ordering of life, alongside the belief in 'historicism' and the maintenance of tradition. The importance of intermediary associations such as the family, community, aid organisations and others in bonding social life and serving in the welfare of people were also supported. Finally, the belief in all of these positive integrating forces were buttressed by a fear of social disorganisation and anxieties over the dissolution of community ties, derived from the liberal-democratic consequences of Revolutionary society in Europe – France in particular – but also from the forces of modernity in general.[17]

The impact of the conservative tradition on Coubertin's philosophy of Olympism, and the manner in which that tradition manifested itself in terms of his eclectic ideals and sources he utilised to support them is far too immense a topic to cover here, but three major foundations, derived from three different epochs, are crucial in understanding Coubertin's wishes and goals for the Olympic movement.[18] Coubertin was inspired by ideals – largely mythologised ones, as it turns out – from ancient, medieval and modern sport. The first and the last have been well documented, but the medieval less so. All three are in fact built into the message to delegates in 1894 cited above, even if they are cloaked in the formal language of his invitation to some degree.

First, in establishing a 'mythology of continuity' between the sporting traditions of antiquity and his proposed modern Olympic movement, Coubertin made his version appear to stand above the crass materialism of industrial capitalism – one of his central goals based on the previously mentioned fears in the nineteenth century conservative movement that influenced him – while simultaneously overcoming the varied amateur conflicts by appealing to a 'universal' form of sport. Unlike the material world of 'advertisement and bluff ... [where] athletic sports are likely to be commercially exploited', Coubertin claimed his Games would 'show beauty and inspire reverence'.[19] Linking the myth of ancient sport as 'pure' was important enough, but Coubertin also sought to combine this imagery while elevating the status of his movement to that of a religion – once again complying with the traditions of European conservatism. The young male athletes of ancient times, Coubertin wrote, 'imbued with a sense of the moral grandeur of the Games, went to them in a spirit of almost religious reverence'.[20] Linking the ancient and religious ideals directly, Coubertin told his audience in a radio broadcast in

Geneva in 1935 that '[t]he primary, fundamental characteristic of ancient Olympism, and of modern Olympism as well, is that it is a *religion*' and that his Games would instil 'a religious sentiment ... [similar to the] religious sentiment that led the young Hellenes, eager for the victory of their muscles, to the foot of the altars of Zeus'.[21] This imagery was powerful and linking modern to ancient sport through religious sentiment successfully enhanced the image of Coubertin's movement as 'pure'.

While the links between modern and ancient sport were powerful and persuasive, the sporting festivals in ancient Greece were vastly different. Rooted in the material conditions of their time, athletes in the ancient games were akin to professional warriors fighting for city-state favours and privilege more so than the 'pure' or 'honourable' ones that Coubertin envisioned. Sport was intimately linked to military training and contests were frequently violent struggles.[22] Also, Coubertin's self-proclamation that he was the regenerator of age-old traditions was somewhat deceitful in a more direct, political sense. Young has demonstrated that Coubertin used other Olympic movements in Greece and England in the mid-to-late nineteenth century as models for his own. Admiring the sporting movement inspired by Englishman William Penny Brookes, whose organisational efforts led to the National Olympic Games held in London's Crystal Palace in 1866, Coubertin never gave Brookes' inspiration for his own Olympic movement its full due. Young points out that 'Coubertin borrowed the ideas of others for his international festival and knowingly declined to give them appropriate recognition'.[23]

Second, the influence of English sport on Coubertin's project was vital. Fashioning himself as an educational reformer in the 1880s, he was sent on fact-finding missions by the French government in the latter years of that decade to North America and the UK. It is well known that Coubertin was influenced by Rugby School headmaster Thomas Arnold and the School's practice of student-run football to instil an admirable blend of masculinity and moral values, alongside the writings of Thomas Hughes (*Tom Brown's School Days*) and Charles Kingsley. The values of Muscular Christianity that Coubertin took from these experiences and works greatly influenced his image for the ideal athlete in the soon-to-be-created Olympic movement. The morally sound athlete was one who embodied duty, courage, honour and self-discipline.[24]

But while the values of the Muscular Christianity movement undoubtedly had a profound influence on his ideals, it was the third epoch – the medieval – and specifically mythologised ideals of chivalry based in prominent writings from the late eighteenth and nineteenth centuries that had a more profound impact, one that has been somewhat overlooked by historians. Indeed, Jeffrey Segrave points out that the muscular Christian athlete personified in the practices of schools such as Eton and Rugby was in Coubertin's mind merely a 'mediator' between his ideals gleaned from a surge of interest in medieval chivalry in France and England and his lofty goals for modern sport.[25] 'True Chivalry', Coubertin wrote, 'existed in only a few scattered individuals without a code, without a fraternal organisation or opportunities and means to help one another, when there appeared in England a century ago these "muscular Christians" among whom one finds in embryo all the qualities of a bygone chivalry – its high ideals, its healthy ruggedness, its generous ardour.'[26]

Three specific values were important in the medieval-based chivalric revival and system of myths in France and England that in turn made their way into Coubertin's set of ideals: honour, loyalty and prowess.[27] Coubertin wrote that '[w]e must establish the tradition that each competitor shall in his bearing and conduct as a man of honour and a gentleman endeavour to prove in what respect he holds the games and what an honour he feels to participate in them'.[28] The ideal of honour manifested itself in important ways in the Games: the rules deciding which men of 'good character or previous record of conduct' should be permitted to participate; the revival of the (ancient and medieval) tradition of taking an oath; and an undying belief in 'fair play' in competition.[29]

In terms of loyalty, Coubertin made the link between knighthood and sport directly, writing that 'elite [athletes] must also be a *knighthood.* ... "brothers in arms", brave, energetic men united by a bond that is stronger than that of mere camaraderie. ... In chivalry, the idea of competition, of effort opposing effort for the love of the effort itself, of courteous yet violent struggle, is superimposed on the notion of mutual assistance, the basis of camaraderie.'[30] Interestingly, the 'spirit of sincere disinterestedness', playing the game for the sheer love of it, derived from a combination of these two ideals of honour and loyalty combined and for Coubertin this spirit was a safeguard against the creeping materialism his project so adamantly resisted.[31]

Finally, prowess represented physical feats in chivalric battle, transposed for Coubertin on to his modern sport movement. But, crucial to these feats was that they be conducted morally or honourably – 'conspicuous moral acts undertaken for the sake of honor rather than utility'.[32] Coubertin certainly admired the physical feats of athletes, but this value-ideal manifested itself in Coubertin's explicitly stated goal that the Olympic athlete in particular would serve as a model for others both in terms of his athletic prowess, and also as a model of behaviour and good conduct. Coubertin invited delegates to his 1894 Congress to consider 'peaceful and chivalrous contests' and it was based on the model of prowess in the chivalric tradition of the nineteenth century that he envisioned his Games.[33]

The codes of knightly conduct that Coubertin so admired were based on idealisations and myths, in a double sense. First, the exploits of the feudal knights from the eleventh to sixteenth centuries in Western Europe upon which the chivalric code was based were idealised in literature. The knights themselves were at times closer to barbaric violent plunderers than the honourable warrior represented in literature.[34] Second, it was the reconstruction of already pre-existing myths in English and French literature in the eighteenth and nineteenth centuries that directly influenced Coubertin's revival of the chivalric tradition in the Olympic movement. Revived chivalric traditions met the needs of conservative empire building and national revitalisation in both countries. For Coubertin, it provided a model upon which to instil 'honourable' values in French youth through a revitalised physical education programme, especially after France's loss in the Franco-Prussian War. Moreover, the particular English resurgence of chivalry that infused itself in the Muscular Christianity movement was the closest and most perfect model of the honourable and virtuous athlete that Coubertin wanted for his movement.[35]

The nature of Coubertin's project, Segrave summarises, was profoundly mythological:

> There was ... no continuous tradition that joined the ancient Olympic Games to chivalry and chivalry to the games of the nineteenth century. Just as the Victorians selected the qualities which they most admired in chivalry and refashioned the cult of games in the light of them, so Coubertin selected the qualities that he most admired in the Arnoldian system and chivalry and created Olympism in their image.[36]

The whole thing was a construction, but a powerful one that satisfied Coubertin's own personal desires for instilling 'honourable' values in the Olympic movement through its most important conduit – the athletes – while simultaneously creating the universalism he needed to fend off competing traditions. It was also a construction that would come to persevere through time and, importantly, frame discussions and policies as Coubertin and the International Olympic Committee (IOC) faced real-world challenges in the early twentieth century. As it turns out, one of the real-world challenges would be 'doping' and its perceived threat to Coubertin's ideals.

Early Twentieth Century Challenges and Nascent Anti-Doping

For the Olympic movement to last, Coubertin and the IOC had to concern themselves from the start with a combination of external challenges, the most notable of which included: existing sporting traditions, the form of which rivalled Coubertin's 'amateur' sport; varied political interests in using the nascent Games for purposes of pursing nation-building agendas; commercial interests in sport, reflecting the wider trend towards treating all aspects of human life as potential commodities; and finally the realities of paying for facilities and generally financing the Games. All of the forces combined were challenges for Coubertin's ideals and the amateur restriction that became the codified expression of those ideals.

For Coubertin, amateur restrictions themselves – whatever form they took – missed the moral and educative goals of his project. Late in his life Coubertin wrote, 'To me, sport was a religion with its church, dogmas, service ... but above all a religious feeling, and it seemed to me as childish to make all this depend on whether an athlete had received a five franc coin as automatically to consider the parish verger an unbeliever because he receives a salary for looking after the church.'[37] Nevertheless, the IOC's first *Bulletin,* published in July of 1894 just after the Paris Congress, formalised the definition of an amateur. Primarily reflecting British amateur definitions based on class traditions and prejudice, the *Bulletin* stated that an athlete could only take part in the Games if he had 'never participated in a competition open to all comers, or competed for a cash prize or a sum of money ... or with professionals – and who has never at any time of his life been a paid teacher or instructor of physical education'.[38] However, formally enforcing this or, for that matter, any amateur rule was difficult for a number of reasons, from basic disorganisation in the movement's first years to complex disagreements about the validity or nature of the amateur restriction. As such, the IOC left enforcement of eligibility mainly up to International Federations for each sport. Indeed, it is known that paid professionals competed in the first few Games in sports such as cycling and fencing, and even the first winner of the marathon in Athens in 1896 received 25,000 drachmas from the Greek government.[39]

The IOC's Charter would eventually formalise eligibility restrictions; however, it would take at least three decades from the start of the movement for the Charter to have any real impact.[40] The first two Olympic Charters of 1908 and 1911 made no mention of amateur restrictions, and while the Charter of 1920 did use the term amateur, it did so not to formally prohibit athletes based on specific principles but, instead, simply as a blanket statement that '[t]he Olympic Games bring together *amateurs* from all nations' and that amateurs needed to be recognised as such by the Olympic committees of their respective country.[41] However, Point 4 of the 1920 Charter is important because, besides requiring that participants be nationals or naturalised citizens of their respective countries and formally recognised by their national Olympic committee, the point ends with the significant sub-clause that athletes be 'd'une honorabilité incontestée'.[42] While there is no perfect English translation, that athletes 'are of a respectability that is beyond reproach' is one strong possibility.[43] However, irrespective of the exact language, the message is clear: the 1920 Charter was attempting to uphold Coubertin's underlying ideal of the chivalric athlete whose honour was absolute.

The 1924 Charter formalised the amateur conditions of participation somewhat, but the conditions merely stated that the amateur status of athletes was to be determined by each respective International Federation, that national federations conform to their parent international counterparts, that in cases in which a sport did not have an international governing body amateur status would be determined by the organising committee of the Games and, finally, that those athletes who were deemed fraudulent would be disqualified.[44] The IOC formalised the amateur code in its Charter more fully in 1930, repeating the conditions of 1924 but adding that as a condition of participation, an athlete: '1. Must not be, or knowingly have become, a professional in the Sport for which he is entered or in any other sport. [and] 2. Must not have received re-imbursement or compensation for loss of salary.'[45] In short, within the first few decades of the twentieth century the IOC had gradually worked out its central principled rule upon which the Olympic movement would be based, even if that rule was far from Coubertin's vision for the ideal 'chivalrous' athlete. This rule and the principles underlying it would, as we will soon see, play a central role in the determination of what constituted an 'ethical' practice or not when doping practices were first debated by the IOC.

The fledging Olympic movement encountered several challenges to Coubertin's ultimate ideals and to the amateur restrictions themselves in the late nineteenth and early twentieth centuries. However, overriding all of these was what Richard Gruneau and Hart Cantelon refer to as the 'universal market' – the commodification of virtually all aspects of human life, including sport and leisure. '[T]he actual possibilities open to [the IOC] were limited by the nature of the economic system as a whole and the network of social institutions associated with it', the authors point out.[46] The tensions between the emerging market economy and the nascent movement took several forms, but a few important examples represent the types of challenges faced.

Officials from Britain, Germany, the USA and Coubertin's own France all resisted the IOC's amateur restriction leading up to the 1896 Games in Athens, feeling they could each best achieve nationalistic goals by entering the best athletes, irrespective of their amateur status. Also, the realities of financing a large event faced the IOC immediately, and without the financing of wealthy businessman George Averoff the ancient stadium where the first modern Games were held would not have been renovated in time.[47] Even the nature of sport itself was highly contested – members of the German Turner Movement and the French Gymnastics Movement supported non-competitive gymnastics such as tumbling, pyramid building and synchronised acrobatics, more so than the English-based competitive sport tradition.[48] The Games, Gruneau and Cantelon continue, were also 'drawn into the economic struggles of modern nation states'.[49] The 1900 Paris, 1904 St. Louis and 1908 London Games were all held in conjunction with international exhibitions celebrating industrial capitalism and modernism, the same forces of materialism – 'an atmosphere of advertisement and bluff' as he put it – that Coubertin blamed for the demise of the great traditions of Europe. Also, despite the IOC's protests, the organisers of the 1928 Amsterdam Games sold rights packages to various companies, including Coca-Cola, permitting them advertising within the stadium and on various buildings in the city.[50]

Perhaps the most important conflict came against the Fédération Internationale de Football Association (FIFA). A sport already greatly professionalised in the early twentieth century and the biggest financial draw for the Games, FIFA proposed a scheme of broken time payments to allow better players and more teams to take part in the Games leading up to the 1928 Amsterdam Games, and the IOC Executive Board voted in favour of such a scheme in 1927, a blatant contradiction of its own rules.[51] Both sides revisited the issue leading up to 1932, but the IOC this time rejected the broken time payments proposal, only to have soccer excluded from the 1932 Los Angeles Games. FIFA countered the move by initiating the World Cup championship in 1930. A compromise was made by 1936, FIFA allowing amateur players into the Games knowing that this move would not threaten its professional status. However, the whole affair pre-shadowed greater – and more systematic – threats to amateurism and, ultimately, to Coubertin's ideals after WWII.[52]

In terms of doping practices and anti-doping policies, most historical work has concentrated on the post-War period when the use of banned substances became a much more common component of athletes' day-to-day training regimens and when, simultaneously, formal regulations alongside sanctions against drugs and proscribed methods were created. However, the recent work of John Gleaves and Paul Dimeo are important because they point out that apprehension about 'doping' at the top levels of Olympic administration date well into the pre-War years.[53] The concerns, it turns out, were directly related to the goals of Coubertin and the defence of amateurism.[54]

Dimeo points out that during the late nineteenth century and the first few decades of the twentieth century, the use of substances and methods that would later become prohibited were, despite some voices of discontent, generally accepted and regarded with an air of curiosity. Alcohol, kola, oxygen and strychnine were used, as were other substances and methods, and historical evidence suggests that attitudes both within athletic circles and in the general public was a mix of support alongside some attempts to control behaviour deemed inappropriate from the perspective of religious temperance.[55] '[T]he science of doping', Dimeo points out, 'developed as a genuine, open and legitimate source of research-based knowledge'.[56] Experimental evidence – derived from studies mainly in Germany, which was ahead of other countries in terms of theoretical research, although research in the USA was also important – was presented in legitimate academic journals on the effects of caffeine, cocaine, sodium phosphate, adrenal hormones, cola nuts and several other stimulants and aids.[57] Stimulants were openly used in professional cycling, pedestrian races and boxing, and amateur rowers, tennis players and runners used alcohol, strychnine, 'purified' oxygen and other substances.[58]

Gleaves has demonstrated that the growing support for the condemnation of doping was very much premised on distinctions regarding what was appropriate or inappropriate behaviour for amateurs versus professionals. The amateur–professional distinction was one that, interestingly, did not exist in the waning years of the nineteenth century and early years of the twentieth century, when the ethics of anti-doping was at best, as Gleaves puts it, 'murky'.[59] However, under a logic that emerged in the first few decades of the twentieth century, 'true' amateur sportsmen would and should never dope, in contradistinction to professional sport, where utilising aids to enhancement was much more readily accepted. Not surprisingly, the line was drawn along class lines: 'Anti-doping rules predicated on amateurism's ideals would simply become another tool for excluding or otherwise marginalising working-class professionals.'[60]

This distinction played a critical role in the first anti-doping rules at the highest levels of organised sport. The International Amateur Athletic Federation wrote in its *Handbook* in 1928 that those known to have doped in 'amateur athletics' could face as much as a lifetime ban.[61] The IOC then made what is believed to be its first statement against the use of 'dope' in 1938, summarising a committee struck the previous year to investigate the matter.[62] The IOC's 1938 *Bulletin* stated: 'The use of drugs or artificial stimulants of any kind must be condemned most strongly, and everyone who accepts or offers dope, no matter in what form, should not be allowed to participate in amateur meetings or in the Olympic Games.'[63] Interestingly, the IOC's first statement against doping in 1938 was spearheaded by staunch amateur defender Avery Brundage, who was also a member of the previously mentioned committee. The IOC would formally enshrine its statement against doping into the Charter in 1946 under 'Resolutions Regarding the Amateur Status'; the anti-doping rule in fact remained as a subset to the Charter's amateur restriction until

1975.[64] Premised on assumptions regarding the 'doped' athlete being contrary to amateurism, then, the IOC would carry its initial restrictions into the post-War era, with all attendant challenges and contradictions.

Cold War Realities: The Death Knell of Amateurism and the Rise of Anti-Doping 'Spirit'

While George Orwell's famous 1945 dictum that sport was becoming 'war minus the shooting' was prescient, he could not know the lengths to which the major players in ensuing cold war rivalries would go to achieve victory and medals on the Olympic stage when he wrote those words.[65] In contrast to Coubertin's wishes that the Olympic movement provide a counter-poise to the 'potent incentive and the dangerous canker' of '[a]thletics for the sake of winning something', the Games in the post-War era quickly grew in status while winning and pursuing athletic superiority through increasingly arduous training regimens quickly made Coubertin's 'honourable' athlete and the moral and educative objectives of sport a thing of the past.[66]

While commercial television and the increasing interests on the part of transnational corporations to use the Olympic Games and its athletes to sell goods and services would eventually put pressures on the IOC to change what was seen as its increasingly antiquated amateur rule, the East–West confrontation between the cold war superpowers was the original catalyst. Although it was decisions made during the 1930s that led the Soviet Union to pursue a high-performance sport system that would compete in bourgeois sport, the actions taken in the post-War period more fully accelerated the USSR's system towards Olympic success. This included a financial rewards system initiated in 1945, an infrastructure to support athletes' training and the use of advanced, scientific training regimes. With the entry of the USSR in the Helsinki Games in 1952, the drama of heightened Olympic cold war competition had formally begun. The partitioning of Germany into east and west only heightened that drama.[67]

Although the pressures to rid the Charter of the increasingly out-of-date amateur restriction were heavy, the IOC maintained the spirit of the amateur clause for three full decades after the end of WWII, with president Avery Brundage (1952–1972) leading the defence. While Swedish delegate Bo Ekelund argued in 1946 that the amateur–professional distinction should be eliminated, Brundage held strong. Reflecting precisely Coubertin's sentiments – and, interestingly, the myths upon which those sentiments were based – Brundage proclaimed that '[t]he amateur code, coming to us from antiquity, contributed to and strengthened by the noblest aspirations of great men of each generation, embraces the highest moral laws. No philosophy, no religion, preaches loftier sentiments'.[68] Also reflecting Coubertin's ideals, the distinction between the amateur and professional, Brundage claimed, 'exists in the heart and not in the rule book'.[69]

Yet, Brundage would defend the 'rule book' much more adamantly than did Coubertin. The 1949 Charter more formally defined an amateur as 'one who participates ... in sport solely for pleasure and for the physical, mental or social benefits he derives therefrom, and to whom participation in sport is nothing more than recreation without material gain of any kind'.[70] Although the language of the amateur rule would change somewhat over the next two decades, the essence of the restriction remained the same. However, During the IOC's meetings in 1967, Soviet delegate Constantin Andrianov pointed out that the amateur clause did not account for the 'requirements of life and conditions in which modern sport is developing' and that 'antiquated formulas of the amateur status' should be renounced.[71] Also, a 1969–1970 IOC–NOC joint commission spearheaded by Romanian delegate

Alexandru Siperco recommended that Rule 26 be changed to the 'Eligibility Code' but, despite the fact that Brundage yielded on the title, the rule itself was if anything more restrictive than ever.[72] Reflecting directly practices that were known to be occurring in the east and west, respectively, the Code specifically banned athletes who were given 'positions in the Army, on the police force, or in a government office' and prohibited 'colleges and universities [that] offer outstanding athletes scholarships and inducements of various kinds'.[73] Expressing his stand in clear terms, Brundage had in fact written to Siperco in 1969: '[w]hy change a system that has operated successfully for sixty years and open the door to outright professionalism?'[74]

By 1974, with Brundage having stepped down, the eligibility restrictions were changed irrevocably. While the 1974 Code still prohibited financial compensation, it permitted assistance under certain conditions, including payments from National Olympic Committees or National Sports Federations, insurance coverage related to training and competition, scholarships and, importantly, '[p]rizes won in competition within the limits of the Rules established by the respective International Federations'.[75] The rule changes were important, first, because the bye-laws now permitted prizes based on international federations' rules and increasingly many of those federations had strong incentives, including direct financial ones, to permit professionals in their competitions. Second, the IOC had yielded on the term 'amateur', an important concession because, as Beamish points out, '[t]erminology plays a crucial role in the struggle over ideas, because words and concepts channel passions and aspirations'.[76] Finally, and related to the previous point, while the amateurism restriction – whatever form it took – was not the most important thing for Coubertin, by the 1970s it was the last connection to Coubertin's ideals. The 'chivalrous athletic effort' of 'honourable' athletes and the 'glittering dream of ancient Olympism' were now gone. 'The IOC had adapted its Charter', Beamish and Ritchie conclude, 'so that the Games would feature the best athletes in the world for whom sport was a full-time, year-round occupation. Winning and the conquest of the linear record were the new foundation of the Olympic Movement'.[77]

In terms of anti-doping, while changes to the Charter's eligibility requirements had moved the Olympic movement more in line with the realities of high-performance sport and the pursuit of record performances, anti-doping prohibitions and, more importantly, the reasons underlying those prohibitions, looked back in time. While many cite the death of Danish cyclist Knud Jensen during the 1960 Rome Games and rumours that he died from an overuse of amphetamines as the central catalyst in the IOC's post-War struggle against doping, Gleaves points out that the foundation for reactions to his death was 'set in motion long before Jensen ever climbed on a bicycle'.[78] The sentiment that began before the War – that amateurs participated in 'pure' sport without the use of aids, while professionals abused 'dope' – only grew in the post-War environment. Immediately after Jensen's death, Gleaves reports that the coach of French cycling defended his team: 'many pros [in France] are drugged, of course, but we won't drug amateurs'. Dr Albert Hyman, former president of the American College of Sports Medicine, expressed a similar condemnation of doping in amateur, but not professional, sport, stating that the professional 'may employ any means which will permit him to achieve his best performance' when he 'has a job to do which may be his sole livelihood'.[79]

Even before Jensen's death spearheaded amateur leaders into action, American J. Kenneth Docherty wrote in the IOC's *Bulletin* that 'our present code of amateurism could never bless such all-out efforts' represented by athletes' use of drugs but pointed out that committing full time to training regimes was also contrary to amateur ideals.[80] At the highest ranks of the IOC, the condemnation of doping along amateur–professional lines was slow, even if, as Gleaves demonstrates, consistent. Brundage was far more concerned with preserving the general principles of amateurism and his view of Coubertin's legacy. Doping was just one subset of a more general principle. Thomas Hunt has also shown that a surprising level of disorganisation alongside disagreements within the organisational hierarchy of the Olympic movement – the IOC itself, International Federations, National Olympic Committees and other groups – hampered strong anti-doping action both before and after drugs were formally prohibited.[81] Brundage mentioned the problem of athletes using 'Amphetamine Sulfate' in IOC meetings in San Francisco in 1960, although the discussion led to little action. Ironically, the same Swedish delegate Bo Ekelund who had called for a reconsideration of the amateur clause in the Charter in 1946 called, in the same 1960 meeting, for a serious investigation of the matter of doping; however, his request was ignored.[82]

With Jensen's death, Brundage and the IOC Executive Board met 15 days later and expressed displeasure with the incident, although mainly from the perspective of public relations; Brundage, who was particularly displeased that Jensen had been awarded a gold medal posthumously, organised in 1962 a doping sub-committee headed by Sir Arthur Porritt, head of the Royal College of Surgeons of England. Hampered by disorganisation and Porritt's ambivalence towards the issue, Brundage replaced Porritt with Dr Ferreira Santos, under whose direction the sub-committee published a statement in the IOC's *Bulletin* in 1963 defining doping as 'an illegal procedure used by certain athletes, in the form of drugs; physical means and exceptional measures which are used by small groups in a sporting community in order to alter positively or negatively the physical or physiological capacity of a living creature, man or animal in competitive sport'.[83] The statement was hampered by quite obvious inaccuracies and vagueness – problems that would continue to hamper anti-doping in the years to come – combined with no formal sanctioning power.[84]

After limited tests on cyclists during the Tokyo Games in 1964 and his regaining the position as head of the sub-committee after Santos's death, Porritt asserted a strong position during the 1965 IOC general meetings in Tokyo, stating that the IOC should issue a formal – and more carefully worded – statement against drugs, create sanctioning procedures and include a promissory clause athletes would have to sign as a condition of participation.[85] Porritt presented a report in April 1966 that included a list of banned substances which would be prohibited at the upcoming 1968 Mexico City Games, highlighting the fact that in his opinion, 'only a long-term education policy stressing the physical and moral aspects of the drug problem would stop athletes from using drugs'.[86] At its Tehran meetings in May 1967 the IOC defined doping formally, voted to add drug and sex testing and to require athletes to sign a pledge to the effect that they do not use drugs. Doping was defined as 'the use of substances or techniques in any form or quantity alien or unnatural to the body with the exclusive aim of obtaining an artificial or unfair increase of performance in competition'.[87]

Dimeo has demonstrated that the decisions made by members of the IOC during the heady years between the death of Jensen in 1960 and the decision to formally ban drugs in 1967 were ones made by men heavily influenced by ideals of sport from a previous age. The fanatical and proselytising approaches some of the earliest and most important anti-dopers took in the post-War period, Dimeo demonstrates, 'were a subtle and implicit – but enormously powerful – force in setting the framework for anti-doping in the 1960s'.[88] Dimeo's analysis is important, first, because he points out that those who crusaded against drugs gradually but systematically shifted the emphasis from one of concern with the health of athletes to a moral emphasis on the character of users and their 'evils'.

Second, the anti-doping movement sought to return sport to its mythical original state. 'Anti-doping was an exercise of power in which the authorities had to protect sport: that meant disseminating the myth of its purity.'[89]

Brundage, the most adamant defender of amateurism, had in fact reduced the drug issue to a secondary place in the list of Olympic problems; it was yet one more piece of evidence that sport had moved further away from Coubertin's original goals. Porritt, writing an article in the *Olympic Review* in 1965 with the simple title 'Doping', reflected Dimeo's points perfectly. Combining his attack on the moral character of users alongside a defence of the Olympic movement's original ideals, Porritt informed his readers that drug users have 'weakness of character' and 'an inferiority complex', and that 'it behoves every one of us interested in the basic values of amateur sport to keep this matter under the closest surveillance and to remember always that the "dope" in the American sense – the mentally, physically and morally dulled individual – is to some degree at any rate the inevitable corollary of doping'.[90] Reiterating the same combination of sentiments, Dr G.M. Oza from India wrote two pieces in the same journal in 1969 and 1971 – 'Athletes, Doping and Olympism' and 'The Olympic Ideal Faces Extinction' – in which he expressed the concern that 'dope' threatened amateur ideals. Citing the amateur rules directly alongside the athletes' oath, Oza stated explicitly that doping is 'not in keeping with the Olympic ideals' because dope is used 'to deprive [an athlete] of sensibility', 'never provides the real pleasure' and 'deprives the athletes of their natural feelings and actions' such that they 'may become lazy and indifferent towards leading the life of a sportsman'.[91]

The dissolution of the amateur rule was consistent with the performance demands that had systemically become an essential component of Olympic competition by the early 1970s. Olympic sport and Olympic athletes were different in kind – not just by degree – from what it/they had been in Coubertin's time. However, the inclusion of the anti-doping sanctions harked back to Coubertin's mythological 'purity' in sport. Expressing this point succinctly, Beamish notes that the rules were 'intimately tied to Coubertin's original lofty principles, and indeed, the use of performance-enhancing substances was, within that context, cheating. ... [However] [o]nce the Olympic Games' fundamental principles were removed, the IOC's most principled rationale for a banned list vanished'.[92]

Conclusion

Foundation myths have been crucial to the survival of the Olympic movement – they were as important in Coubertin's time as they are today. But while the particularities of the myths that were evoked depended on the various political expediencies of the day, underlying it all was the myth that the Olympic movement represented a universal and pure form of sport. Resorting to an extreme teleological historicism – one of the foundations of conservatism summarised by Beamish earlier – Coubertin wrote in 1896 that the Olympic revival 'is not the result of a spontaneous dream, but the logical consequence of the great cosmopolitan tendencies of our times'.[93] Coubertin, Segrave summarises, 'was able to rationalize and popularize his Olympic project as the teleological destination of an identifiable world-historical process'.[94] 'His' modern Games, in other words, were not a human reinvention, but the natural culmination of history marching towards its inevitable perfection. But Coubertin's 'honourable' and 'chivalric' athlete was never possible because he never existed in the first place. However, amateurism – the tradition that came closest to satisfying Coubertin's lofty goals while allowing him to achieve practical political objectives during the movement's nascent days – became the movement's cherished principle. As the IOC faced the challenges of enhanced competition, sportive nationalism, commercialism and, as it turns out, doping in both the pre- and post-War decades, the defence of amateurism only grew stronger but more desperate.[95] But while Coubertin's ideals gradually faded further into history and while the amateur restriction as the formal representative of those ideals fought its last fight in the late 1960s and early 1970s, anti-doping prohibition looked back to both amateurism and, ultimately, Coubertin for its justification.

Currently, there are many who defend the legitimacy of the 'spirit of sport' clause in the World Anti-Doping Agency's *Code*, including philosophers who defend the ethical premises of the clause in its current or perhaps slightly modified form.[96] Also, there are of course other important reasons for the creation of anti-doping policies in the Olympic movement beyond the 'spirit of sport'; in particular, the concerns regarding the health of athletes and the principle of fairness in sport have and continue to be legitimate concerns. However, the important point raised here is that amateurism and, ultimately, Coubertin's 'sport mythology' should not be discounted because they played a crucial role. The 'political history' of the modern Olympic movement, Stephen Wagg points out, 'has entailed a dialogue with the ghost of the movement's chief founder'.[97] The particular political dialogue summarised here – the dialogue the IOC has had with certain performance-enhancing substances and methods – continues to be a dialogue with Coubertin as well.

Today, the movement requires a continued notion that it represents 'pure' sport and that it continues to be 'something else'. While there are a number of ways this is accomplished – ceremonies, the oath, symbols, the torch relay and others – the specific role that anti-doping plays in perpetuating Olympic sport's 'essence' is one of the most important. Currently, the various agents who premise anti-doping regulations on the 'spirit of sport' may not believe that their campaign is based on long-standing ideals about the essence or purity of sport that harken back to Coubertin. They may not, in other words, believe that the policies they have constructed are based on mythology. But of course, in founding his Olympic movement, neither did Coubertin.

Notes on Contributor

Ian Ritchie is Associate Professor in the Department of Kinesiology at Brock University, St. Catharines, Ontario, Canada.

Notes

1. World Anti-Doping Agency, *World Anti-Doping Code,* 14.
2. There are several accounts of the mythology of 'purity' and 'timelessness' of the modern Olympic Games; see, for example, Rider and Wamsley, "Myth, Heritage"; or Beamish and Ritchie, *Fastest, Highest, Strongest.* Other accounts of this mythology are referred to throughout this article.
3. De Coubertin, *Olympism,* 543. Originally published as "Why I Revived the Olympic Games" in *Fortnightly Review* July (1908): 110–5.
4. David Young's work is the most important: Young, *The Olympic Myth;*Young, "How the Amateurs Won", "From Olympia 776BC."
5. Kidd, "Another World in Possible," 146. See also Kidd, "The Myth."
6. It should be pointed out at this point that the argument here applies specifically to the spirit of sport clause of the *World Anti-Doping Code,* and not the other two main criteria used to warrant inclusion of substances or methods in the *Code's* list: fairness and the health. These two other criteria have each played their own important roles in terms of justifying anti-doping policies historically.

7. See Guttmann, *The Olympics,* 7–20 on these various challenges. Also, see DaCosta for an excellent summary of attempts to define the philosophy of 'Olympism' from Coubertin's day up to the present: DaCosta, "A Never-Ending Story."
8. Slater, "Modern Public Relations"; Chatziefstathiou, "Pierre de Coubertin: Man and Myth"; Chatziefstathiou, "The History of Marketing."
9. MacAloon, *This Great Symbol,* 194; Guttmann, *The Olympics,* 14; de Coubertin, *Olympism,* 308–12.
10. Cited in MacAloon, *This Great Symbol,* 194.
11. Ibid.
12. De Coubertin, *Olympism,* 300–2; Young, "How the Amateurs Won," 65.
13. De Coubertin, *Olympism,* 305.
14. Cited in Young, "How the Amateurs Won," 74, note 22.
15. De Coubertin, *Olympism,* 301. Originally printed as a circular letter, "Cirulaire Annonçant le Congrès International Athlétique," Paris, January 15, 1894.
16. Spencer, "The Nature of Society," 140.
17. Beamish, *Steroids,* 7–10.
18. The literature on Coubertin is immense, although a few sources can be highlighted: Coubertin, *Olympism,* is, as far as I know, the largest collection in English of Coubertin's writings and speeches, while MacAloon's *This Great Symbol* is considered the quintessential biography of Coubertin. See also: Beamish, *Steroids,* 1–24; Beamish and Ritchie, *Fastest, Highest, Strongest,* 11–30; Beamish and Ritchie, "From Chivalrous"; Guttmann, *The Olympics,* 7–20; Chatziefstathiou, "Pierre de Coubertin"; Chatziefstathiou, "The History of Marketing"; Segrave, "Coubertin, Olympism, and Chivalry"; Young, *The Olympic Myth;*Young, "How the Amateurs Won"; Young, "From Olympia 776BC"; Young, *A Brief History.*
19. De Coubertin, *Olympism,* 543, 545. Originally published as "Why I Revived the Olympic Games" in *Fortnightly Review* July (1908): 110–5.
20. Ibid., 543.
21. Ibid., 580.
22. See Kidd, "The Myth"; Young, "From Olympia 776BC"; Spivey, *The Ancient Olympics.*
23. Young, "From Olympia 776BC," 16.
24. Brown, "The Olympic Games Experience," 22–3. See also Wagg's excellent general description of amateurism: Wagg, "Tilting at Windmills."
25. Segrave, "Coubertin, Olympism, and Chivalry," 20. Dr Segrave's paper was presented at the 11th International Symposium for Olympic Research in London, Canada, October 19, 2012, under the title 'Modern Olympism as Medieval Knight: The Transubstantiation of Chivalry in Coubertin's Ideology of Olympism'. However, Dr Segrave provided me with a full-length article upon which the presentation was made. The full-length article is under the title cited here. As far as I am aware, the article is the most comprehensive analysis of Coubertin's ideal of medieval chivalry. I am grateful to Dr Segrave for providing his copy of this article.
26. Cited in Ibid., 20–1.
27. Ibid., 23–29.
28. De Coubertin, *Olympism,* 546. Originally published as "Why I Revived the Olympic Games" in *Fortnightly Review* July (1908): 110–5.
29. Segrave, "Coubertin, Olympism, and Chivalry," 23–5. The quotation regarding character and conduct is from Coubertin: De Coubertin, *Olympism,* 546.
30. De Coubertin, *Olympism,* 581. Originally from a radio broadcast by Coubertin in Geneva, August 4, 1935, and published as "Les Assises Philosophiques de l'Olympisme Moderne" in *Le Sport Suisse* 37 (7): 1.
31. Segrave, "Coubertin, Olympism, and Chivalry," 26–7. The quotation regarding the spirit of disinterestedness is from Coubertin: De Coubertin, *The Olympic Idea,* 15. The original is from "Letter to Charles Simon" published in *Revue Olympique*, July 1906.
32. Ibid., 28.
33. Ibid. Coubertin's words are from de Coubertin, *The Olympic Idea,* 2. The original is from a circular letter of January 15, 1894, published in *Bulletin du Comité International des Jeux Olympiques*, July 1894.
34. Ibid., 5–8.
35. Ibid., 10–21.
36. Ibid., 21.

37. De Coubertin, *Olympism,* 654. The original was published in Coubertin's *Olympic Memoirs,* Chapter 11, held in the IOC Archives in Lausanne, Switzerland. Regarding the various forms that amateurism took, Richard Gruneau points out that 'the IOC formed committee after committee to study the meaning of amateurism and try to define it in practical terms'. Gruneau, "'Amateurism' as a Sociological Problem," 573.
38. Cited in Beamish, "Pierre de Coubertin's Shattered Dream," 491. The bulletin is also available in the original French through the LA84 Foundation website: http://www.la84foundation.org/OlympicInformationCenter/RevueOlympique/1894/BCIF1/BCIF1e.pdf (accessed April 26, 2013). For discussions of the influence of British sport on the Olympic codification of amateurism, see Wagg, "Tilting at Windmills"; Gruneau, "'Amateurism' as a Sociological Problem"; Young, "How the Amateurs Won."
39. Wagg, "Tilting at Windmills," 324.
40. See Teetzel, "Charting the Charter."
41. Comité International Olympique, *Charte Olympique,* 1920: 8–9, http://www.olympic.org/olympic-charters?tab=1 (accessed April 27, 2013). On the 1908 and 1911 Charters, see Comité International Olympique, *Charte Olympique,* 1908 and 1911, http://www.olympic.org/olympic-charters?tab=1 (accessed April 26, 2013).
42. Ibid., 9.
43. I am grateful to Dr Leslie Boldt for translations and nuanced commentary regarding the language used for this clause in addition to other sections of the Charters from 1908 to 1924 that are available in French only.
44. Comité International Olympique, *Charte Olympique,* 1924: 12–13, 18. http://www.olympic.org/olympic-charters?tab=1 (accessed April 27, 2013).
45. Comité International Olympique, *Charte Olympique,* 1930: 24. http://www.olympic.org/olympic-charters?tab=1 (accessed April 27, 2013). Llewellyn and Gleaves point out that this language came from IOC meetings in 1925 and specifically the debate within the IOC whether to accept broken time payment schemes, especially in football. Llewellyn and Gleaves, "The Rise of the 'Shamateur'," 23–4, 28 note 7.
46. Gruneau and Cantelon, "Capitalism, Commercialism, and the Olympics," 352.
47. Guttmann, *The Olympics,* 15–6.
48. Ibid., 16–17.
49. Gruneau and Cantelon, "Capitalism, Commercialism, and the Olympics," 353.
50. Barney, Wenn, and Martyn, *Selling the Five Rings,* 28–9. Coubertin's comment on advertising is from De Coubertin, *Olympism, 543.*
51. Llewellyn and Gleaves, "The Rise of the 'Shamateur'," 23–4.
52. Beamish and Ritchie, *Fastest, Highest, Strongest,* 16–7.
53. Gleaves, "Doped Professionals"; Dimeo, *A History of Drug Use.*
54. Gleaves, "Doped Professionals."
55. Dimeo, *A History of Drug Use,* 17–50.
56. Ibid., 33.
57. Ibid., 35–42.
58. Gleaves, "Doped Professionals," 242–246. Hoberman's *Mortal Engines* traces the birth of doping back to the original development of relationships formed between biomedical scientists and athletes in the late nineteenth century when scientists were interested in discerning biophysiological 'truths' about the human body. However, performance enhancement – doped or otherwise – was not the goal of scientists at the time. Hoberman is less specific about the creation of the first anti-doping rules.
59. Gleaves, "Doped Professionals," 243.
60. Ibid., 241.
61. Ibid., 238, 246, 251 note 6.
62. *Official Bulletin of the International Olympic Committee,* 1937, 6. Lausanne: International Olympic Committee. Accessed through the LA84 Foundation website: http://www.la84foundation.org/OlympicInformationCenter/OlympicReview/1937/BODEb35/BODEb35b.pdf (accessed April 29, 2013). See also the more detailed history of this statement and the IOC's policies more generally in the Gleaves and Llewellyn article published in the current volume.
63. *Bulletin Officiel du Comité International Olympique, 1938,* 30. Lausanne: International Olympic Committee. Accessed through the LA84 Foundation website: http://www.la84foundation.org/

OlympicInformationCenter/OlympicReview/1938/BODEb37/BODEb37d.pdf (accessed April 29, 2013).

64. This information comes from the work of Gleaves and Llewellyn in the article contained in the current volume. The IOC resolved to include the anti-doping statement in the Charter in 1938 but it was not included until 1946 because the War interrupted the Charter's production.
65. Orwell, "The Sporting Spirit," 198.
66. Beamish and Ritchie, *Fastest, Highest, Strongest.* Beamish and Ritchie also point out that the ontology of training changed in the post-War era, from an emphasis on 'fixed capacities' to expanding potentials. See Beamish and Ritchie, "From Fixed Capacities" and *Fastest, Highest, Strongest*, 52–59. Coubertin's comment is from De Coubertin, *Olympism, 543.*
67. There are several sources on this history, but in terms of the relationship between accelerated cold war competitions and doping, see Beamish and Ritchie, *Fastest, Highest, Strongest,* 17–30, 66–104; Beamish, *Steroids,* 41–72; Dimeo, *A History of Drug Use,* 53–86. See also, Dennis and Grix, *Sport Under Communism,* for a careful consideration of the German Democratic Republic's sport system. On the specific point about the Soviet Union's decision in the 1930s, see Beamish, *Steroids,* 43–5.
68. Cited in Guttmann, *The Games Must Go On,* 116.
69. Ibid.
70. International Olympic Committee, *Charter of the Olympic Games,* 1949: 18. http://www.olympic.org/olympic-charters?tab=1 (accessed April 29, 2013).
71. Cited in Beamish and Ritchie, *Fastest, Highest, Strongest,* 25.
72. Siperco has an interesting history in the Olympic movement. See Ionescu and Terret, "A Romanian Within the IOC," and specifically pp. 1183–85 on his role in the joint commission. I am also indebted to Richard Pound's commentary on the importance of Siperco in the amateur debate within the ranks of the IOC. Personal interview with Richard Pound, Toronto Canada, January 14, 2013. The interview was part of a separate research project being conducted by the author.
73. International Olympic Committee, *Charter of the Olympic Games,* 1971: 48. http://www.olympic.org/olympic-charters?tab=1 (accessed April 29, 2013).
74. Cited in Ionescu and Terret, "A Romanian Within the IOC," 1183.
75. International Olympic Committee, *Charter of the Olympic Games,* 1974: 13–4. http://www.olympic.org/olympic-charters?tab=1 (accessed April 29, 2013).
76. Beamish, "Pierre de Coubertin's Shattered Dream," 498.
77. Beamish and Ritchie, *Fastest, Highest, Strongest,* 28.
78. Gleaves, "Doped Professionals," 250. Møller points out that Jensen died of heatstroke and extreme dehydration and not amphetamine use. Møller, "Knud Enemark Jensen's Death." Also, a critique of the notion that anti-doping started with Jensen is the main focus of the Gleaves and Llewellyn article published in the current volume.
79. Both cited in Gleaves, "Doped Professionals," 250.
80. Cited in Dimeo, *A History of Drug Use,* 96.
81. Hunt, *Drug Games.*
82. Ibid., 10.
83. Cited in Ibid., 15.
84. Ibid.
85. Ibid., 17.
86. Ibid., 22–3. See also Beamish and Ritchie, *Fastest, Highest, Strongest,* 21.
87. Cited in Todd and Todd, "Significant Events," 68.
88. Dimeo, *A History of Drug Use,* 95.
89. Ibid., 119–20.
90. Porritt, "Doping," 47–9.
91. Oza, "Athletes, Doping and Olympism." See also Dimeo, *A History of Drug Use,* on Oza's 1971 article. Oza's points are instructive and historically relevant because his two articles were published in *Olympic Review*. However, it is not clear what role Oza played in the Olympic movement, nor does Dimeo discuss his relevance in any general sense.
92. Beamish, *Steroids,* 71.
93. De Coubertin, *The Olympic Idea,* 10. The original is from *Les Jeux Olympiques 776 av. J.-C – 1896.* Edition grecque-française: Athènes/Paris, Ch. Beck/H. Le Souldier (1896): 1–7.
94. Segrave, "Coubertin, Olympism, and Chivalry," 4.

95. 'Sportive nationalism' is an expression that has been used widely to refer to sport competition for national aggrandizement, but as far as I know the expression was originally John Hoberman's. See Hoberman, "Sport and Ideology."
96. Notably, see Loland and Hoppler, "Justifying Anti-Doping"; McNamee, "The Spirit of Sport."
97. Wagg, "Tilting at Windmills," 321.

References

Barney, R. K., S. R. Wenn, and S. G. Martyn. *Selling the Five Rings: The International Olympic Committee and the Rise of Olympic Commercialism*. Salt Lake City: The University of Utah Press, 2002.

Beamish, R. "Pierre de Coubertin's Shattered Dream." *Queen's Quarterly* 103, no. 3 (1996): 488–501.

Beamish, R. *Steroids: A New Look at Performance-Enhancing Drugs*. Santa Barbara, CA: Praeger, 2011.

Beamish, R., and I. Ritchie. *Fastest, Highest, Strongest: A Critique of High-Performance Sport*. New York: Routledge, 2006.

Beamish, R., and I. Ritchie. "From Chivalrous 'Brothers'-in-Arms' to the Eligible Athlete: Changed Principle and the IOC's Banned Substance List." *International Review for the Sociology of Sport* 39, no. 4 (2004): 355–371.

Beamish, R., and I. Ritchie. "From Fixed Capacities to Performance-Enhancement: The Paradigm Shift in the Science of 'Training' and the Use of Performance-Enhancing Substances." *Sport in History* 25, no. 3 (2005): 412–433.

Brown, D. A. "The Olympic Games Experience: Origins and Early Challenges." In *Global Olympics: Historical and Sociological Studies of the Modern Games*, edited by K. Young and K. B. Wamsley, 19–41. Amsterdam: Elsevier JAI, 2005.

Chatziefstathiou, D. "The History of Marketing an Idea: The Example of Baron Pierre de Coubertin as a Social Marketer." *European Sport Management Quarterly* 7, no. 1 (2007): 55–80.

Chatziefstathiou, D. "Pierre de Coubertin: Man and Myth." In *The Palgrave Handbook of Olympic Studies*, edited by H. J. Lenskyj and S. Wagg, 26–40. New York: Palgrave Macmillan, 2012.

DaCosta, L. "A Never-Ending Story: The Philosophical Controversy Over Olympism." *Journal of the Philosophy of Sport* 33 (2006): 157–173.

De Coubertin, P. *The Olympic Idea: Discourses and Essays*. Stuttgart: Carl-Diem-Institut, 1967.

De Coubertin, P. *Olympism: Selected Writings*. Lausanne: International Olympic Committee, 2000.

Dennis, M., and J. Grix. *Sport Under Communism: Behind the East German 'Miracle'*. New York: Palgrave Macmillan, 2012.

Dimeo, P. *A History of Drug Use in Sport 1876–1976: Beyond Good and Evil*. London: Routledge, 2007.

Gleaves, J. "Doped Professionals and Clean Amateurs: Amateurism's Influence on the Modern Philosophy of Anti-Doping." *Journal of Sport History* 38, no. 2 (2011): 237–254.

Gruneau, R. "'Amateurism' as a Sociological Problem: Some Reflections Inspired by Eric Dunning." *Sport in Society* 9, no. 4 (2006): 559–582.

Gruneau, R., and H. Cantelon. "Capitalism, Commercialism, and the Olympics." In *The Olympic Games in Transition*, edited by J. O. Segrave and D. Chu, 345–364. Champaign, IL: Human Kinetics, 1988.

Guttmann, A. *The Games Must Go On: Avery Brundage and the Olympic Movement*. New York: Columbia University Press, 1984.

Guttmann, A. *The Olympics: A History of the Modern Games*. 2nd ed. Urbana, IL: University of Illinois Press, 2002.

Hoberman, J. *Mortal Engines: The Science of Performance and the Dehumanization of Sport*. New York: The Free Press, 1992.

Hoberman, J. "Sport and Ideology in the Post-Communist Age." In *The Changing Politics of Sport*, edited by L. Allison. Manchester: Manchester University Press, 1993.

Hunt, T. M. *Drug Games: The International Olympic Committee and the Politics of Doping, 1960–2008*. Austin: University of Texas Press, 1960.

Ionescu, S. A., and T. Terret. "A Romanian within the IOC: Alexandru Siperco, Romania and the Olympic Movement." *The International Journal of the History of Sport* 29, no. 8 (2012): 1177–1194.

Kidd, B. "'Another World Is Possible': Recapturing Alternative Olympic Histories, Imagining Different Games." In *Global Olympics: Historical and Sociological Studies of the Modern Games*, edited by K. Young and K. B. Wamsley, 143–158. Amsterdam: Elsevier JAI, 2005.

Kidd, B. "The Myth of the Ancient Games." In *Five Ring Circus: Money, Power and Politics at the Olympic Games*, edited by A. Tomlinson and G. Whannel, 71–83. London: Pluto Press, 1984.

Llewellyn, M. P., and J. Gleaves. "The Rise of the 'Shamateur': The International Olympic Committee and the Preservation of the Amateur Ideal." In *Problems, Possibilities, Promising Practices: Critical Dialogues on the Olympic and Paralympic Games* (Proceedings of the 11th International Symposium for Olympic Research), edited by J. Forsyth and M. K. Heine, 23–28. London: The International Centre for Olympic Studies, 2012.

Loland, S., and H. Hoppeler. "Justifying Anti-Doping: The Fair Opportunity Principle and the Biology of Performance Enhancement." *European Journal of Sport Science* 12, no. 4 (2012): 347–353.

MacAloon, J. J. *This Great Symbol: Pierre de Coubertin and the Origins of the Modern Olympic Games*. London: Routledge.

McNamee, M. J. "The Spirit of Sport and the Medicalisation of Anti-Doping: Empirical and Normative Ethics." *Asian Bioethics Review* 4, no. 4 (2012): 374–392.

Møller, V. "Knud Enemark Jensen's Death during the 1960 Rome Olympics: A Search for Truth?" *Sport in History* 25, no. 3 (2005): 452–471.

Orwell, G. "The Sporting Spirit." In *Shooting an Elephant and Other Essays*, 195–199. London: Penguin, 2003.

Oza, G. M. "Athletes, Doping and Olympism." *Olympic Review* April, no. 19 (1969): 209–212.

Porritt, A. "Doping." *Olympic Review* 90 (1965): 47–49.

Rider, T. C., and K. B. Wamsley. "Myth, Heritage and the Olympic Enterprise." In *The Palgrave Handbook of Olympic Studies*, edited by H. J. Lenskyj and S. Wagg, 289–303. New York: Palgrave Macmillan, 2012.

Segrave, J. O. "Coubertin, Olympism, and Chivalry." Paper presented at the 11th International Symposium for Olympic Research, London, Canada, October 19–20, 2012.

Slater, J. "Modern Public Relations: Pierre de Coubertin and the Birth of the Modern Olympic Games." In *The Global Nexus Engaged: Past, Present, Future Interdisciplinary Olympic Studies* (Proceedings for the Sixth International Symposium for Olympic Research), edited by K. B. Wamsley, R. K. Barney, and S. G. Martyn, 149–160. London, Canada: International Centre for Olympic Studies, 2002.

Spencer, H. "The Nature of Society." In *Theories of Society: Foundations of Modern Sociological Theory*, Vol. I, edited by T. Parsons, E. Shils, K. D. Naegele and J. R. Pitts, 139–143. New York: The Free Press of Glencoe, 1961.

Spivey, N. *The Ancient Olympics*. Oxford: Oxford University Press, 2004.

Teetzel, S. "Charting the Charter: An Analysis of the Eligibility Rules and the Olympic Games." *Olympika* 20 (2011): 31–54.

Todd, J., and T. Todd. "Significant Events in the History of Drug Testing and the Olympic Movement: 1960–1999." In *Doping in Elite Sport: The Politics of Drugs in the Olympic Movement*, edited by W. Wilson and E. Derse, 65–128. Champaign, IL, 2001.

Wagg, S. "Tilting at Windmills? Olympic Politics and the Spectre of Amateurism." In *The Palgrave Handbook of Olympic Studies*, edited by H. J. Lenskyj and S. Wagg, 321–336. New York: Palgrave Macmillan, 2012.

World Anti-Doping Agency. 2009. "World Anti-Doping Code." Accessed April 22, 2013. http://www.wada-ama.org/Documents/World_Anti-Doping_Program/WADP-The-Code/WADA_Anti-Doping_CODE_2009_EN.pdf

Young, D. "From Olympia 776 BC to Athens 2004: The Origin and Authenticity of the Modern Olympic Games." In *Global Olympics: Historical and Sociological Studies of the Modern Games*, edited by K Young and K. B. Wamsley, 3–18. Amsterdam: Elsevier JAI, 2005.

Young, D. C. *A Brief History of the Olympic Games*. Malden, MA: Blackwell, 2004.

Young, D. C. "How the Amateurs Won the Olympics." In *The Archaeology of the Olympics: The Olympics and Other Festivals in Antiquity*, edited by W. J. Raschke, 55–75. Madison: The University of Wisconsin Press, 1988.

Young, D. C. *The Olympic Myth of Greek Amateur Athletics*. Chicago: Ares, 1984.

Sport, Drugs and Amateurism: Tracing the Real Cultural Origins of Anti-Doping Rules in International Sport

John Gleaves and Matthew Llewellyn

Department of Kinesiology, California State University, Fullerton, USA

The historiography of doping has focused primarily on anti-doping efforts that followed in the wake of Knud Enemark Jensen's death in 1960 and culminated in the first Olympic anti-doping tests in 1968. Such focus has often led to the mistaken claim that prior to 1960, the International Olympic Committee (IOC) had not banned doping, and, more importantly, ignores the cultural origins of anti-doping that took hold prior to the Second World War and which shaped the IOC's response to doping following Jensen's demise. By tracing early doping practices through turn-of-the-century horse racing and its concerns over gambling and the interwar efforts to ban doping in Olympic sports through the amateurism code, the authors examine the influences behind the IOC's decision to first ban doping in 1938. More importantly, it roots the post-Jensen anti-doping rhetoric and legislation in the early twentieth-century push to defend amateurism against the perceived nefarious forces of gambling, commercialism, professionalism and totalitarianism that were supposedly overrunning amateur sport in the 1930s.

Introduction

In the late summer of 1960, the world's athletes gathered for the Rome Olympic Games. Few anticipated that these Games would forever change international sport. The unseasonably warm weather challenged many athletes as the mercury regularly passed 30°C. In the men's cycling 100 km team time trial, the oppressive heat proved too much for the four-man Danish cycling team. After one lap of Rome's Via Cristoforo Colombo, Jørgen Jørgensen, dropped out due to sunstroke. Needing three riders to finish in order for their time to count, Niels Baunsøe, Vagn Bangsborg and Kund Enemark Jensen persevered. When shortly thereafter Jensen complained of dizziness, Baunsøe and Bangsborg took hold of the cyclist, both pushing and supporting their fading teammate. Tragedy soon struck when Jensen collapsed to the ground and fractured his skull. Being unconscious, an ambulance transported Jensen to an overheated military tent, where he soon passed away.[1]

Jensen's death – the first ever in an Olympic Games – reverberated around the world. With much of the sporting press in Rome to cover the Games, media outlets quickly seized upon the tragedy. The story would take an unexpected twist when Oluf Jorgensen, the

Danish cycling team's trainer, admitted to providing Jensen and his teammates with Roniacol, a drug used to reduce blood pressure. Although the autopsy listed heatstroke as the official cause of death, no doubt exacerbated by his head trauma, media reports somewhat dubiously linked Jensen's demise to doping.[2] The International Olympic Committee (IOC) took Jensen's death as a call to action and implemented an organised effort to prevent doping which the IOC maintained until it helped establish and fund the independent World Anti-Doping Agency in 1999.[3]

Placing this unbroken line with Jensen provides historians with a neat starting point to examine anti-doping efforts in sport. Indeed, much of the doping literature focuses on the period following Jensen's demise as the point where sporting organisations started taking the issue of doping seriously. Historian Thomas Hunt uses Jensen's death in 1960 as his starting point in *Drug Games: The International Olympic Committee and the Politics of Doping, 1960–2008*.[4] The doping scholar Ivan Waddington dates 'the introduction of anti-doping regulations' to the 1960s.[5] To a certain extent, evidence supports such focus. In the years following Jensen's death, the IOC established a medical commission to examine doping (1962), implemented drug testing (1968) and suspended its first athlete, the Swedish pentathlete Hans-Gunnar Liljenwall, for doping violations (1968).[6] Thus it is undeniable that much of today's legislative and bureaucratic anti-doping efforts point back to Jensen and the increased concern about doping in the years after his death. But much of the prevailing historiography ignores earlier anti-doping efforts. Others have gone one step further, erroneously asserting that prior to Jensen's drug-related death no anti-doping rules existed at the Olympic Games. The doping scholar Verner Møller writes that when Jensen and his teammates used Roniacol, 'doping was not illegal at the time'.[7] Historian Paul Dimeo even goes so far as to conclude that as late as 1964, within the Olympic Games 'no rules had yet been established against doping'.[8]

The general historical emphasis on post-Jensen anti-doping is shortsighted, as bureaucratic efforts to stamp out the practice existed for six decades prior to the Dane's demise – the IOC executive committee prohibited doping as early as 1938 and even introduced the ban as part of Rule 26 in their next published charter in 1944 where it stayed until well into the 1970s.[9] The IOC was not alone in establishing early anti-doping legislation: The International Amateur Athletic Federation (IAAF) prohibited doping in 1928.[10] While in the sport where doping first occurred, horse racing, efforts to eliminate the practice date to the nineteenth century.[11] Such a myopic focus also largely ignores the intellectual framework that governed the IOC's nascent efforts to combat doping in sport.[12] Rather than viewing anti-doping initiatives as a coordinated medical response to the tragic death of an Olympic cyclist in 1960, an alternative history reveals that bureaucratic concerns about doping not only predated the Second World War but were also framed by the IOC almost exclusively within the context of amateurism. As the IOC's regulatory framework governing conduct and eligibility, amateurism required athletes uphold certain moral standards. The Olympic amateur played the game for the game's sake, disavowed gambling and professionalism, and competed in a composed dignified manner fitting of a 'gentleman'.[13] Anti-doping rhetoric, and later legislation, first emerged as part of the early twentieth-century push to defend amateurism against the perceived nefarious forces of gambling, commercialism, professionalism and totalitarianism that were supposedly overrunning amateur sport.

These previously ignored anti-doping efforts as well as the intellectual framework that inspired them matter because they shaped the IOC's response to doping in the years after Jensen's drug-related death. In fact, these early anti-doping attitudes continue to subtly shape the contemporary anti-doping discourse that governs sport today. Tracing the real cultural origins of anti-doping through horse racing's early discourses and later the IOC's decision that doping violates the amateur sporting ethos reveals how the twin pillars of anti-doping – that the practice is unhealthy and unsporting – took hold as popular tropes now common to contemporary sporting culture.

The Origins of Doping

Doping is fundamentally a product of post-enlightenment modern sport.[14] That is not to say that ancient Greek athletes or medieval jousters never ingested substances hoping to gain an edge – surely some charlatan could be found hawking magic potions or promoting a new ingredient outside of the stadium in Olympia. Doping, however, was a product of the Scientific Revolution. As historian Allen Guttmann has pointed out, the post-Enlightenment application of scientific principles to sport marked a Copernican revolution from traditional to modern sport. As traditional sport gave way to modern practices of rational recreation in the mid-nineteenth century, athletes began rationalising their sporting performances. They used scientific methods to improve their training and incorporated modern technological advances to assist them in their sporting endeavours. Along with quantifying and recording athletic records, by the mid-nineteenth century athletes sought to apply scientific standards to training and competing.[15] Horse trainers used watches to time intervals and boxers studied anatomy to expose their opponents' weaknesses.[16]

This rationalised approach naturally led people to explore the burgeoning fields of physiology, medicine and pharmacology – which after all captured the age's *zeitgeist* – for substances that could alter physical performances. Trade with Asia, Africa and South America had introduced a number of stimulants to Western Civilisation including the kola nut, opium and cocaine.[17] By 1889, the use of drugs to alter performance had become known by the verb form 'doping', taken from an earlier noun which meant 'a stupid person'.[18] The sport of kings, horse racing, had long proven itself an early adopter of modern sporting principles.[19] Thus it is no surprise that it would be the first to embrace pharmacological substances to alter horses' performances and it is also from this sport that the word 'doping' was first used to refer to a substance intended to *modify* athletic performance.[20] As Gleaves has argued elsewhere, it is important to emphasise 'modify' when discussing horse racing – and in fact most early accounts of doping – because unlike current connotations of doping, at least through the 1930s doping practices often intended to *harm* athletic performances.[21] In horse racing, trainers would often dope a horse to make it run slower in order to profit from betting on fixed races.[22] Similarly, human athletes would occasionally accuse a trainer of doping them if they performed unexpectedly poor. In either case, doping was usually done to assist shady gambling practices.[23]

For this reason, early opponents of doping emerged from the horse racing ranks and rejected doping not out of any high-minded ideal about the spirit of sport but out of the practical need to ensure fair betting at the tracks.[24] As early as 1903, tracks and horse racing organisations created the first rules banning doping in any sport.[25] The rhetoric, which flooded popular newspapers around the start of the twentieth century, spoke harshly of those responsible for doping horses because it allowed them to swindle other members of the gambling community.[26] The major issue was not drugs so much as the fixing of matches. Press accounts and reactions from those within the horse racing community labelled doping the 'greatest threat to the sport' and such rhetoric continued well into the 1930s.[27]

In human events, the use of stimulants occurred simultaneous to their adoption in horse racing, although they were not met with the same immediate disapproval.[28] Endurance athletes competing in long-distance pedestrian and cycling races at the turn of the twentieth century sought substances to ward off fatigue, experimenting with readily available elixirs including coffee and tobacco.[29] By the start of the twentieth century, common stimulants included alcohol, cocaine, caffeine, opium, strychnine and digitalis.[30] While not all of these substances actually had the effects intended by the athletes – in many instances, the substances likely harmed performance – the post-enlightenment desire to rationalise and enhance human performance drove interest in the burgeoning pharmacological arts.[31]

Curiously, doping was not met with the same degree of moral disapproval in human sports as it was in horse racing, most likely because as John Hoberman points out, 'this early doping was not regarded as an illicit practice; it was rather seen as an antidote to the extreme fatigue experienced by the elite athletes of that era.'[32] Nonetheless, objections to doping with stimulants still emerged. In an 1899 article titled 'The Greatest Athlete That Ever Lived', the author praised 'the foremost of American athletes' and 'a model amateur', William B. Curtis, for abstaining from stimulants and maintaining a pure lifestyle of an amateur athlete.[33] At the collegiate level, both the Harvard and Yale crew teams made a similar point in 1900 by forbidding their athletes from using stimulants during the season.[34] In a 1901 article in *Women's Physical Development*, author J.C. Burns described how 'gymnastics and athletic exercises have lately become generally recognized as being far superior to the "drug treatments" so long in vogue.'[35] Setting healthy sport against 'doping the patient' exemplifies the general belief that 'drugs' and 'healthy living' inherently conflicted with one another. In 1905, the Christian newspaper *Herald of Gospel Liberty* pointed to the use of strychnine in American football as evidence of the sport's immoral influences.[36]

Despite such objections, many voices at the start of the twentieth century expressed few moral qualms about using stimulants.[37] An 1895 article in the *New York Times* acknowledged that professional athletes could use such drugs 'in order to help them prepare for their work', but that no 'true athletes' (a veiled synonym for amateur athletes) would use 'any such injurious and adventitious aids'.[38] While such sentiment would later influence the IOC's decision to prohibit doping, not every amateur athlete shared the *New York Times*' opinion. Indeed, the Cambridge University graduate and amateur tennis champion Eustace White boasted in 1901 that 'alcohol does have certain advantages for modern athletic conditions'. White believed that when a player felt tired near the end of a tennis match and needed 10 more minutes of good play, 'he takes a glass of brandy; he keeps up for ten minutes longer; he wins'.[39] A person considered at that time to be a model amateur athlete, White's attitude towards stimulants indicated that he did not see any conflict with the values of amateur sport. Moreover, White reveals other amateur athletes used alcohol for training purposes. To ward off 'staleness', White explains, the Cambridge crew team would take a glass of port following training and a beer at midday.[40] *The Times* dates the use of alcohol for training back to an 1860 resolution from the Oxford rowing team stating that it would pay for the champagne it deemed necessary for the athletes' training.[41]

Nonetheless, turn-of-the-century professional sport proved much more accepting of drugs. In part, the *de facto* class-divide separating working-class professionals and gentleman amateurs allowed professional athletes the freedom to use stimulants free from amateur sport's 'moralising' influence. Professional sports such as boxing, pedestrianism and cycling openly permitted athletes to use stimulants as needed from the 1890s to the 1910s.[42] The old problem of doping athletes to lose still remained an issue. Professional cycling trainer James 'Choppy' Warburton allegedly used substances to prevent one of his athletes from winning a race, although many professional cyclists switched to his care in order to use his legendary elixirs. By 1903, the public's expectation that professional athletes put on a good show increased to the point that in one case, a reporter openly lamented the lack of doping when fatigue slowed the riders at a 6-day cycling race at New York City's Madison Square Garden. The journalist complained that 'some of them seemed sadly in need of stimulants.'[43] A 1904 article discussed the value of 'a good second' – the person who works in the prizefighter's corner – during a prizefight since they knew how to 'dope the boxers with stimulants'.[44]

The grinding nature of professional sports such as cycling and prize fighting where pay was moderate and performance-based meant newspaper reports portrayed stimulants as a tool to assist professional athletes in doing their job.[45] The general sentiment towards stimulants – as opposed to the doping used to fix horse races – did not see doping as unfair or cheating but simply contrary to the gentlemanly amateur code that governed middle- and upper-class sport. When undertaken by members of the working classes, the act of doping to assist in physical labour fits within the acceptable social behaviours. From the vantage of their 'social betters', the professional need to use stimulants to support their arduous labours reaffirmed the assumed class striations along the manual labour divide. For the 'lower classes', sport was not a means of leisure but a means for economic profit and entertainment. Using sport for such purposes precluded these individuals from realising the middle- and upper-classes notions about sport's moral purpose. Indeed, the tacit tolerance of doping in professional sport permitted upper class social groups to delegitimise the professional athletic performances among those from less powerful social status.

Such tensions were clearly displayed at the Olympic Games. Baron Pierre de Coubertin's vision of the Olympic Games and his tacit embrace of amateurism often put him at odds with the ideology's true advocates, especially on the issue of stimulants. As historian John Hoberman explains:

> De Coubertin's creation of the modern Olympics thus coincided with the early phase of sports medicine that included informal testing of less toxic substances such as milk, tea, and alcoholic beverages. While it is conceivable that de Coubertin could have read about such experimentation in the 1894 volume of the *Archives de physiologie normale et pathologique,* there is no evidence that he did. De Coubertin did, however, anticipate the consequences of the Olympic motto *citius, altius, forties* ('faster, higher, stronger'), and he did so without the trepidation of today's anti-doping activists. De Coubertin knew that the modern sport for which he had created an international stage possessed an element of what he called 'excess'. 'We know', he said in 1901, 'that [sport] tends inevitably toward excess, and that this is its essence, its indelible mark.'[46]

Coubertin's fascination with excess and his comfort with professional sport were clearly displayed in endurance sports such as the cycling races and, his personal initiative, the Olympic marathon. Many viewed the marathon as not really an amateur sport; entrants in the marathon often emerged from the working classes with hopes of parlaying their Olympic fame into lucrative professional contracts. Given this background, it is no surprise that in both 1904 St Louis and the 1908 London Olympic marathons, the use of doping featured prominently. In 1904, the American runner Thomas Hicks, on his way to winning Olympic gold, used a combination of strychnine, egg whites and brandy without anyone objecting to his doping.[47] Four years later while leading the 1908 Olympic marathon, the Italian marathoner, Dorando Pietri, stumbled and struggled towards the finish line. Newspaper reports document how, in order to assist the brave runner, doctors administered stimulants three times.[48] Adding to that, one of the track officials who assisted Pietri, Maxwell Andrews, reported that a Dr Daniel Bulger had witnessed Pietri take 'a dope of strychnine and atropia' during the race.[49] Interestingly, the Italian was later disqualified from the marathon not as a result of his use of dope, but rather because of the unfair assistance offered by British officials when carrying his flagging body across the finishline. Despite his disqualification and open use of stimulants, Queen Alexandria of Great Britain presented the Italian with a special silver cup for his display of bravery and perseverance. Even Baron Pierre de Coubertin, labelled Pietri the 'moral winner of the competition', an odd statement when viewed against contemporary attitudes towards doping.[50]

Most likely, Hicks' and Pietri's use of stimulants in the marathon raised little concern for those seeking to preserve amateur sport since the anti-doping advocates realised that these athletes never qualified as true 'gentleman amateurs' and fell outside the moral code of amateur sport. Moreover, given the strenuous and time-consuming nature of the marathon, the event itself always carried professional overtones for the amateur ideologues. While prior to their Olympic races neither Hicks nor Pietri had competed for pay or raced against professionals, most people understood that these types of athletes intended to turn pro if the opportunity arose and that the values of amateurism never truly applied to the two runners.[51] In the case of Pietri, the Italian later made the switch from the amateur to the professional ranks and allegedly continued his use of stimulants throughout his successful pedestrian career.[52]

These athletes illustrate how working-class professionals (or amateurs viewed as soon-to-be professionals from the working classes) did not see sport in the same moralised manner as middle-class amateurs. This disagreement between the two classes at times caused frustration. Often one such place was cycling's pre-eminent race, the Tour de France, where the desires of the middle-class managers and boosters to promote a socially acceptable spectacle butted up against the habits of working-class professionals. In one incident, where professional cyclists Henri Pelissier, Francis Pelissier and Maurice Ville abandoned the Tour de France in protest of the conditions in the 1924 race, they sat down at a café with journalist Albert Londres, from the French newspaper *Le Petit Parisien.* Londres recorded their conversation:

> 'We suffer on the road. But do you want to see how we keep going? Wait ... '
>
> From his bag he takes a phial. 'That, that's cocaine for our eyes and chloroform for our gums ... '
>
> 'Here', said Ville, tipping out the contents of his bag, 'horse liniment to keep my knees warm. And pills? You want to see the pills?' They got out three boxes apiece.
>
> 'In short', said Francis, 'we run on dynamite'.[53]

The working-class connotation of Londres' 'convicts of the road' epitomises the widely accepted doping culture amongst professional cyclists in France. Historian Christopher Thompson explains that working-class behaviour, such as doping, often led to tensions with Henri Desgrange, the creator of the Tour de France, who expected cyclists to behave in more socially acceptable ways. Yet evidence exists that with professional cyclists, their working-class behaviour often endeared them to their fans, much to the frustration of upper management.[54]

By the 1920s, general social views towards drugs shifted. In Great Britain, the patrician classes increasingly articulated that the working classes should not be permitted to use drugs since they lacked the moral fortitude to stave off addiction – ironically, the upper classes sanctimoniously engaged in frequent drug use on the grounds that they were 'morally superior'.[55] In sport, however, the converse was true. The public widely permitted the use of doping – the same substances the working classes could not use for recreational enjoyment – in professional sports in much the same way that they tolerated gambling and violence. For those concerned with defining middle-class leisure through amateurism, the behaviour of the working classes for whom honour and chivalry were absent from their sporting code only served to reinforce their belief that their place in the social order was well deserved. Thus when members of the IOC chose to address the doping issue, a number of professional and amateur issues shaped their subsequent decisions.

Objections to Doping Take Root

In the aftermath of the Great War, the growing prevalence of doping in competitive sport aroused considerable concern amongst amateur sporting officials. The IOC spearheaded the bureaucratic fight against doping, framing their opposition within the context of amateurism. The inter-war transformation of the Olympic Games into a highly politicised, nationalistic, global sporting festival heightened the regularity of amateur violations. The expanding global and commercial dimensions of the Olympics presented amateur athletes with increased opportunities to parlay their sporting talents into economic reward. Under-the-table 'black money', padded-expense accounts, extended training camps and broken-time payments – monetary compensation to help defray for time away from the workplace – became a common trend within amateur sporting circles. Fearing the transformation of the Olympic Games into a 'shamateur' event, an emboldened IOC, in conjunction with its affiliated international and national sports federations, was determined to get tough. Idealism had to be governed and enforced. Athletes who transgressed Olympic amateur rules were to be punished.[56]

At the same time, many of the IOC's amateur policies coalesced to support the view that doping contradicted the amateur sporting ethos. For example, despite early efforts to eradicate drug use in horse racing to preserve fair gambling environments, doping – and the concerns about fixed races – persisted throughout the 1920s. Newspapers frequently reported doping scandals at unscrupulous tracks. The continued association with gambling placed doping practices directly at odds with the IOC's long-held amateur ethos that forbade gambling as well as the old patrician way of practicing sport rejected by the new amateur.[57] In fact, the nascent IOC determined at its Olympic Congress in 1894, held in Paris, that betting on sport, in any sense, was incompatible with their understanding of amateurism.[58] Furthermore, the muscular Christianity and the temperance movements increased their influence on amateur sport in the USA and Great Britain. This influence meant that by the late 1920s, certain factions within the IOC would scarcely entertain the earlier behaviour of runners such as Hicks or Pietri or cyclists imbibing 'stimulants' of brandy or whisky along the race route. The now widely known doping practices of professional cyclists, footballers and pugilists by the start of the 1920s left few doubting where doping fell on the professional/amateur divide. So in the midst of fighting back against those tarnishing the spirit of amateurism, the sporting world took aim at doping.[59]

Against this backdrop of gambling, drinking and professionalism, international sporting bureaucracies began crafting anti-doping legislation beginning in 1928 with the IAAF – an organisation founded and led by Sigfrid Edström, a devout amateur apostle and high-ranking Olympic official. During its 9th Congress held in Amsterdam on July 27 and continuing through August 6–7, 1928, the IAAF crafted a new round of stringent amateur policies designed to stem the tide of semi-professionalism flooding amateur sport. Mr Jean Genet of France captured the anti-professional sentiment of the Congress in his report on appearance fees:

> Before the coming menace, before the bad examples ... given in other sports, before the vexations concessions, in my opinion, made by the IOC with reference to the "deficit not earned", we have the duty of carefully studying the situation, of making the texts stricter if necessary, and of completing them by very clearly worded formulas that will make it clear to all our adherents that we are Amateurs [sic] in the full sense of the word, and that we intend to remain Amateurs [sic].[60]

Aside from prohibiting broken-time payments and appearance fees – emerging trends in amateur track and field throughout Europe and North America – the IAAF chose to make their 'texts stricter' by passing rules banning doping. The IAAF executive council, having studied the question of doping at sessions held during the 1928 Olympic Games in Amsterdam, proposed to the Congress on August 6 'that a rule should be made prohibiting the use of drugs or stimulants in athletic competitions'.[61] With a unanimous vote, the Congress's 74 delegates representing 28 countries agreed 'that such a rule should be introduced, whereupon a lively discussion ensured as to the text to be adopted in this respect', with various propositions and amendments handed to the executive council to be transferred into definite text. The next day, the Council proposed the following text to its Congress:

> Doping is the use of any stimulant not normally employed to increase the power of action in athletic competition above the average. Any person knowingly acting or assisting as explained above shall be excluded from any place where these rules are in force or, if he is a competitor, be suspended for a time or otherwise, from participation in amateur athletics under the jurisdiction of this Federation.[62]

Despite the IAAF's trail-blazing anti-doping efforts, its formative definition of what actually constituted doping proved as malleable and troublesome as the definition of amateurism. Reporting to British expatriates on 'home sport', a special correspondent to Singapore's *Straight Times* wrote that the IAAF's ban on doping 'is very right and proper, but they have not supplied any definition of what "doping" is, and until they do so, their edict cannot have very much practical effect'.[63] Illustrating the confusion, the author pondered:

> Does half a glass of brandy before a race amount to dope, or is it only other drugs than alcohol that are aimed at? Some of the later, such as strychnine, are far more insidious in their effects, and far more liable to cause permanent harm, than sherry or spirits, and in the professional world, mixtures containing them are far from unknown.[64]

Although failing to clearly define doping, the IAAF's passage of an anti-doping rule generated little global media attention. While the *New York Times* briefly acknowledged that the IAAF had breached the doping issue, it proved more concerned about American sprinter Charley Paddock's eligibility for the upcoming Amsterdam Games.[65] In Great Britain, *The Times*, the *Guardian* and the *Observer* all ignored the IAAF's landmark piece of legislation. The Edinburgh *Scotsman* did make brief note of the topic, commenting that although 'rare in Great Britain', and 'heartily condemned by sportsmen in this country', the IAAF had 'issued a ban the practice of 'doping' athletes prior to a race'.[66] Melbourne's daily *Argus* was the only Australian newspaper to mention the IAAF's new rule, writing that 'The federation, for the first time, recognized doping as an existing fault, and made provisions for the exclusion of any person knowingly doping or assisting in doping.'[67] Considering the global prominence that doping bans would later take, it is surprising that so little was made of the IAAF's nascent anti-doping efforts.

While the IAAF never appeared to have used this rule to ban any athletes or trainers, in other sports, accusations of doping did emerge. Following the 1932 Olympics Games in Los Angeles, U.S. swim coaches levelled doping charges at members of the Japanese men's swim team which had surprisingly trounced their American counterparts, winning gold in five of the six races. After the Games, two U.S. swim coaches, Matt Mann and

Robert Kiphuth, formed a National Collegiate Athletic Association subcommittee to investigate allegations that the Japanese swimmers breathed purified oxygen prior to their events. Mann adamantly denounced the actions of the Japanese men as doping (despite no rules prohibiting the practice) and declared a 'war against doping' of amateur swimmers, such as was done by the Japanese in the 1932 Olympic Games. Moreover, Mann sought rules 'to forestall the danger of the practice spreading in this country, as it was unethical, regardless of harmful effects'.[68]

Mann's accusations that doping amateur swimmers with oxygen was unethical, regardless of health effects, likely included nationalistic motives. Following a public drubbing, Mann desired to delegitimise the performance of the Japanese. The Associated Press' sports editor, Alan Gould, noted as much in his criticism of Mann:

> It seems quite all right, in principle to conduct a 'war against doping' in the matter of star swimmers or athletes in general, but it smacks of poor sportsmanship at this date for any American, much less a college coach, to belittle the magnificent victory of Japan's young swimmers in the 1932 Olympics, on the basis that oxygen was used by them as a stimulant.

Gould subsequently called Mann's criticism of doping 'altogether inopportune and out of order', pointing out the legacy of American use of stimulants in past Olympic sports.[69]

Mann's comments – and Gould's response – indicate the larger cultural forces at work. Mann's nationalist criticism would not have resonated with newspaper reporters nor the general public – nor would Mann have even offered doping as criticism – unless the general public already believed that doping contradicted amateur values. By tenuously tying the Japanese swimmers to the practice of doping, Mann marginalised the swimmers' accomplishments. Gould's reaction reveals this effect, as he attempted to restore credibility to the Japanese swimmers, calling them 'grand sportsmen', and asserting that 'the Japanese would have won the Olympic swims, anyway, with or without [oxygen]'.[70] Mann intended his criticism of the Japanese to resonate with a broader audience – an audience that also perceived doping as un-amateur and undesirable. Mann and Gould's interchange reveals that a general climate existed that viewed doping as incongruent with amateurism. These views indicate, at least partially, that the wider public also likely accepted a similar narrative during the inter-war years.

The IOC Gets Involved

Although the alleged use of stimulants by Japanese swimmers at the 1932 Los Angeles Games did not spark an immediate reaction, it was not long until the IOC addressed doping. Following the infamous 1936 Olympic Games in Berlin, complaints emerged that the Nazi's and a host of fellow authoritarian right-wing regimes had openly flouted the IOC's existing rules on amateurism. Reports of state-run training camps and sizable governmental subsidies for amateur athletes prompted IAAF president (and newly appointed IOC vice-president) Sigfrid Edström to suggest the formation of a new IOC to investigate these allegations.[71] In preparation for this committee, IOC president Henri de Baillet-Latour drafted an essay 'upon various points figuring on the Agenda of the coming Meeting in Warsaw', under the heading: 'AMATEURISM'.[72] In this essay, Baillet-Latour listed seven immediate questions on amateurism that need to be addressed, including 'Doping of Athletes'. The wealthy former Belgian racecourse owner opined:

> amateur sport is meant to improve the soul and the body therefore no stone must be left unturned as long as the use of doping has not been stamped out. Doping ruins the health and very likely implies an early death.

He concluded by asking 'What do you propose?'[73]

Extensive archival research indicates that this statement by Baillet-Latour is the first recorded comment by an IOC official on the issue of doping. Baillet-Latour, who had owned several racehorses and been president of the Jockey-Club Bruxelles, was likely first introduced to the doping issue through his time in the horseracing world.[74] Jockey Clubs around the world had battled doping throughout the 1910s and 1920s. Baillet-Latour's essay on amateurism, however, not only placed doping within the context of amateurism, much like the IAAF in 1928 and Matt Mann did in 1932, but also made it one of the central concerns for the IOC to address at its 1937 Congress in Warsaw, Poland. At that meeting, members of the IOC's executive board opened their June 9 morning session to a number of amateur issues. While shifting through allegations of 'shamateurism' and authoritarian extended training camps, British IOC member Lord David Burghley (the Marquess of Exeter) raised the importance of studying the 'doping of athletes'.[75] The IOC promptly formed a special commission comprising some of its most distinguished officials: Sweden's Sigfrid Edström, American Avery Brundage, Italian Count Alberto Bonacossa and German Karl Ritter Von Halt.[76] Of these four, both Edström and Brundage would serve as IOC presidents and were undoubtedly the most ardent promulgators and defenders of Olympic amateurism. Von Halt served as the president of the organising committee for the Fourth Winter Olympic Games and would go on to direct the Sports Office of the Third Reich before leading the German Olympic Committee from 1951 to 1961.[77] Certainly, this was no 'back-water' committee.

Although Burghley broached the subject, few within the IOC including Baillet-Latour had previously done anything to address the doping issue. In a 1937 letter to Paul Anspach, president of the International Fencing Federation, IOC secretary Albert Berdez, wrote that 'on the question of Doping [sic] .... The IOC has no record on the issue.'[78] He also pointed out that president Baillet-Latour claimed to have no personal record on the issue either. Such evidence indicates that the efforts initiated in 1937 were the first anti-doping queries undertaken on the IOC's behalf. Regarding why Baillet-Latour brought up doping, Berdez explained that 'His attention was drawn to this issue by the sounds everywhere on the use of drugs by athletes, including athletics and cycling.'[79] It also likely reflected his deep roots in horse racing, where doping had been an ongoing problem and where he had likely first encountered the issue as an owner of horse racing tracks. In that sense, horse racing, although coincidently, shaped amateur sport once again.

Anspach took Berdez's letter as indication that the IOC needed additional information on doping and thus sent a report on doping in fencing and shooting that indicated a much more sophisticated view on the subject than previously expressed within the IOC.[80] Anspach's attached report was one of many investigations into doping that Baillet-Latour would gather between the IOC's Warsaw meeting in 1937 and its Cairo meeting in 1938. The IOC received additional reports from both the Belgian Medical Society for Physical Education and Sport (SMBPES) and Italian doctor G. Poggi-Longostrevi. Taken together, these reports represented the state of doping in the era before the Second World War. In these early documents, the authors cite two common themes about doping. First, the documents assert that doping was unhealthy. Second, the documents contend that doping does not belong in sport. Galfre's report indicated that the drugs used by athletes posed harm to their organisms by upsetting its normal balance.[81] The SMBPES objected to doping first, 'because it is harmful to health' and second, 'it poisons the atmosphere of sport ... and creates a mentality inconsistent with the true spirit of sportsmanship.'[82] The Italian doctor Poggi-Longostrevi referred to 'deadly stimulants' and advocated Olympic rules that empowered judges who suspect doping 'be permitted to test this athlete by a committee of doctors an objective examination of the athlete's organism and examining secretions and giving the positive results by testing'.[83] Although the substances mentioned in the reports including strychnine, caffeine, alcohol, heroin and the Kola nut are taken for granted by the authors as common doping techniques, only one specific case of doping – the Japanese use of purified oxygen in Olympic swimming in 1932 – is mentioned.

Whether these reports made it back to the IOC's amateurism commission is unclear, but the IOC's decision to archive these reports under 'Amateurism Issues' alongside other issues such as amateurs competing with professionals in ice hockey and paid ski instructors competing as amateur ski racers indicates that IOC clearly considered doping an issue related to amateurism.[84] More importantly, the Olympic officials serving on the committee appeared to share these sentiments. The committee met twice, once in Cologne and later in Paris between the 1937 IOC session in Warsaw and the 1938 IOC session held in March in Cairo, Egypt. Writing sometime between these two meetings, American IOC chief Avery Brundage observed: 'The use of drugs or artificial stimulants of any kind cannot be too strongly denounced and anyone receiving or administering dope or artificial stimulants should be excluded from participation in sport or the O.G. [Olympic Games].'[85] The special commission submitted nearly identical language to Brundage's original handwritten note (only changing 'denounced' to 'condemned' and including 'in any manner' in the final draft) for inclusion in their report delivered during the Cairo session. Thus Brundage, who would be the IOC president at the time of Jensen's death in 1960, had already penned the language that would provide the framework for the IOC's response as early as 1937.

The strong language and relative lack of amendments indicate that IOC members in general shared similar attitudes concerning doping. Compared to the special committee's other topics such as 'question of nationalism for political purposes', and 'the situation of professional journalists', which included numerous amendments and revisions, the 'doping of athletes' garnered little opposition. However, the glaring omissions, such as policies for testing for drugs and detailed policies for enforcing the ban, indicate that although members concurred on the issue, anti-doping was still in its infancy. On March 17, 1938, the IOC adopted a final 10 resolutions on amateurism which would be included in the next Olympic Charter. Although a revised charter would not appear until after the Second World War in 1946, the committee's resolutions, including its statement against doping, appeared unchanged under 'Resolutions Regarding the Amateur Status'.[86] Considering that doping at the Olympic Games would later garner major headlines, little fanfare existed when the IOC passed its first anti-doping rule.[87] The press supplied almost no coverage of the IOC's new resolutions and completely ignored the decision to ban doping. An extensive search of media coverage of sport from 1937 to 1939 did not find a single mention of the IOC's decision to prohibit doping, although admittedly press coverage was more focused on the larger political and military issues appearing on the horizon.

Conclusion: Drugs Without Amateurism

Despite the Second World War's interruption of the Olympic Games, the IOC's decision to ban doping emerged in the next Olympic Charter published in 1946.[88] Far from forgotten, these pre-war resolutions stayed in the Charter as resolutions regarding amateur status. This language would continue as part of Rule 26 – the IOC's rule on amateurism – until 1975, where it was transferred from an eligibility rule to part of the IOC's new 'medical code' with separate bi-laws created by the IOC's Medical Commission. More importantly, the attitudes that justified anti-doping in the years before the Second World

War – that doping was unhealthy and violated sport's amateur ethos – continued to shape anti-doping attitudes throughout the second half of the twentieth century.

In light of the cultural origins of anti-doping legislation in sport, the prevailing historiographical association with Knud Jensen and the 1960s ignores the factors that existed before and at the time of Jensen's death. After all, claims that no rules banning doping existed at the time of Jensen's death are simply wrong. The IOC did have a rule that expressly forbade doping as a criterion for competition which had been accepted as early as 1938. More tellingly, in the years following Jensen's death, the IOC used this pre-existing rule in their charter as a starting point for addressing doping. Rather than inventing a new rule, the IOC simply added, amended and modified the text originally handwritten by Avery Brundage in 1937. In fact, from 1962 through 1975, the IOC's anti-doping rule remained part of the IOC's eligibility rule – the rule governing its amateur requirements – which was its most seriously enforced rule governing athletes' conduct. In that sense, a clear and unbroken legislative link connects the IOC's 1938 ban on doping to its anti-doping efforts throughout the 1960s.

While claims that the IOC had no rules prohibiting doping before 1960 are false, what about the general focus on post-1960 anti-doping efforts? Critics might admit that although the IOC did have a rule prohibiting drugs, it did not begin to seriously address doping until the 1960s, thus focus on this era is justified. But, accurately understanding these actions and the reasons that drove them can only make sense in light of the IOC's earlier efforts. The belief that anti-doping attitudes were products of the 1960s ignores the intellectual foundations put in place decades before. Perhaps it would be more accurate to conclude that while anti-doping policies grew more established in the period following Jensen's death, the intellectual and legislative framework that governed anti-doping's expansion existed decades prior. Arguably, the most accurate reading of the events following Jensen's death is that the IOC, although it had passed a rule prohibiting doping, had failed to act seriously on the issue prior to the tragedy in Rome and that Jensen's death forced Olympic leaders to engage the problem on a meaningful level but that both the legislative and cultural foundations for these efforts were erected in an earlier era.

Such an understanding acknowledges the intellectual origins of anti-doping prior to Rome, but also helps explain the increased efforts that followed Jensen's demise. Although perhaps few on the IOC's amateurism committee anticipated how large the doping issue would eventually become, the desire to preserve amateur sport as a moral sphere of healthy competition would influence sports into the twenty-first century. This is because the doping crises and scandals in the 1960s, 1970s and 1980s played out on the Olympic stage. This forced the IOC, rather than other sporting organisations, to blaze the trail for doping policies. At the same time, the IOC's *de facto* role as the leading bureaucratic organisation for sport meant that its policies and directions often influenced other sporting bodies as well as popular opinion. Once the persistent drip of doping scandals turned into a deluge during the 1990s, the Olympic movement invoked its traditional status as the moral guardians of sport to enforce anti-doping tests and suspensions as a way to keep sport pure.

Note the tremendous irony here. As the IOC moved to keep sport pure by launching a war on doping, they simultaneously dismantled amateurism, the very ideal that gave rise to the issue. By the close of the millennium, most Olympic sports permitted professional athletes to compete in the Game. At the same time, anti-doping attitudes had never been higher. In that sense, elements of amateurism still live on in the Olympic Games today. Though no longer seeking to enforce amateurism's code, the IOC still helps ensure athletes to still follow amateurism's moral tenets by enforcing anti-doping rules in sports.

Notes on Contributors

John Gleaves is an Assistant Professor at California State University, Fullerton, CA, USA.

Matthew Llewellyn is an Assistant Professor at California State University, Fullerton, CA, USA.

Notes

1. For a fuller discussion of Jensen, see Møller, "Knud Enemark Jensen's Death."
2. Ibid.
3. This is still the version of events presented on the World Anti-Doping Agency's website. See WADA, "A Brief History of Anti-Doping." Accessed June 6, 2013. http://www.wada-ama.org/en/about-wada/history/.
4. Hunt, *Drug Games*, ix.
5. Waddington and Smith, *Introduction to Drugs in Sport*, 8 and 18.
6. Dimeo, *History of Drug Use in Sport*, 96, 99 and 114.
7. Møller, "Knud Enemark Jensen's Death," 465.
8. Dimeo, *History of Drug Use in Sport*, 103.
9. International Olympic Committee, "The Olympic Charter, 1944," International Olympic Committee Olympic Studies Centre, Quai d'Ouchy, 11001 Lausanne, Switzerland (hereafter cited as IOC Archives).
10. International Amateur Athletic Federation, Annual Meeting Minutes, 1928, IOC Archives.
11. See Gleaves, "Enhancing the Odds."
12. Gleaves, "Doped Professionals and Clean Amateurs."
13. For a more complex treatment of amateurism, see Llewellyn and Gleaves, "Rise of the Shamateur."
14. Hoberman, *Mortal Engines.*
15. Guttmann, *From Ritual to Record.*
16. Ibid.
17. Davenport-Hines, *Pursuit of Oblivion.*
18. Indeed, the vast majority of times doping was used in connection to horse racing and sport and not the general drugging of people, see 'Dope, V[1]', In *Oxford English Dictionary.* Oxford University Press, 1989.
19. For a fuller treatment of modern sport, see Guttmann, *From Ritual to Record.*
20. For more on horse racing, see Gleaves, "Enhancing the Odds."
21. Ibid. Any specific pages for any of these?
22. Ibid.
23. Ibid.
24. Ibid.
25. "'Dope' Evil of the Turf" (*New York Times*, October 19, 1903).
26. Gleaves, "Enhancing the Odds."
27. Ibid.
28. For the dating and introduction of stimulants to human events, see Hoberman, *Mortal Engines.*
29. Dimeo, *History of Drug Use in Sport.*
30. Ibid.
31. Bahrke and Yesalis, *Performance-Enhancing Substances in Sport and Exercise.*
32. Hunt, *Drug Games*, ix.
33. "Greatest All Around Athlete That Ever Lived" (*Fort Worth Morning Register*, July 16, 1899).
34. "College Muscle: Uncle Sam Seeks Suitable Diet and Analyzes Foods Consumed by Harvard and Yale Crews" (*The Biloxi Daily Herald*, April 18, 1900).
35. J.C. Burns, "Casting Out Devils" (*Women's Physical Development*, November 1, 1900).
36. "Foot-Ball" (*Herald of Gospel Liberty*, December 14, 1905).
37. "'Doping' of Athletes" (*The Times*, July 18, 1953).
38. "The Use of Stimulants by Athletes" (*New York Times*, December 1, 1895).
39. Eustace White, "Athletes and the Effect of Alcohol" (*The State*, June 28, 1901), 6.
40. Ibid.
41. "'Doping' of Athletes" (*The Times*, July 18, 1953).
42. "Brooklyn Prize Fighting" (*New York Times*, August 28, 1894) and "The Use of Stimulants by Athletes" (*New York Times*, December 1, 1895).

43. "Cyclist Behind Record" (*New York Times*, December 9, 1903).
44. "Seconds of Pugilists Often Win a Battle" (*The National Police Gazette*, January 2, 1904).
45. "Cyclists Ride to Keep Lead" (*New York Times*, December 10, 1904).
46. Hunt, *Drug Games*, ix.
47. Dyreson, *Making the American Team* and Llewellyn, "'Viva L'Italia! Viva L'Italia!'," 89.
48. Dimeo, *History of Drug Use in Sport*, 28.
49. Ibid.
50. Muller, *Pierre De Coubertin*, 72.
51. Both Hicks and Pietri would capitalize on the pedestrian craze and go on to successful professional running careers, see Llewellyn, "'Viva L'Italia! Viva L'Italia!'."
52. For a fuller treatment of Pietri's professional career, see ibid.
53. Thompson, *Tour de France*, 190.
54. Ibid.
55. For a fuller treatment of this thesis, see Davenport-Hines, *Pursuit of Oblivion*, 61–98.
56. For more on the growing commercialism of the Olympics during the interwar period, see Barney, Wenn, and Martyn, *Selling the Five Rings*.
57. Holt makes this point in a recent talk on amateurism, see Holt, "Origins of Amateurism in Victorian Britain."
58. 'Summary Report, 1894–1930', Box 77, Folder 'IOC meetings', Avery Brundage Archives, University of Illinois Archives, 901 West Illinois Street, Urbana, Ill, 61801 (hereafter cited as Brundage Archives).
59. Gleaves, "Doped Professionals and Clean Amateurs."
60. International Amateur Athletic Federation, Annual Meeting Minutes, 1928, Section 17, Report by Mr Genet of France, 'appearance money', IOC Archives, 43.
61. Ibid., 39.
62. Ibid., 55.
63. "Home Sport" (*The Straight Times*, September 6, 1928).
64. Ibid.
65. "Parade of Athletes Will Mark Opening of Olympics Today" (*New York Times*, July 28, 1928).
66. "Use of 'Dope'" (*The Scotsman*, August, 9 1928).
67. "Olympic Games" (*The Argus*, August 9, 1928).
68. "Charges Japanese 'Doped' Swimmers" (*New York Times*, January 14, 1933).
69. "Sport Slants" (*The Gettysburg Times*, January 24, 1933).
70. Ibid.
71. International Olympic Committee, Meeting of the Executive Committee, Berlin, July 31. 1936, IOC Archives.
72. Henri de Baillet-Latour, 'Essay on Amateurism' (undated but probably 1937) Box 44, Folder 'Baillet-Latour Letters', Brundage Archives.
73. Ibid.
74. Findling and Pelle, *Encyclopedia of the Modern Olympic Movement*, 435.
75. International Olympic Committee, Annual Meeting Minutes, IOC Session, Warsaw, June 9, 1937, IOC Archives.
76. Ibid.
77. Kruger, "Role of Sport in German International Politics."
78. Albert Berdez to Paul Anspach, October 12, 1937, ID Chemise: 204766 CIO COMMI-ADMIS 1935–1967, IOC Archives.
79. Paul Anspach to Albert Berdez, November 6, 1937, ID Chemise: 204766 CIO COMMI-ADMIS 1935–1967, IOC Archives.
80. Report, Dr E. Galfre, 1937 'Du Doping', ID Chemise: 204766 CIO COMMI-ADMIS 1935–1967, IOC Archives.
81. Ibid.
82. Report, undated, 'Rapport Sur le Doping', ID Chemise: 204766 CIO COMMI-ADMIS 1935–1967, IOC Archives.
83. Report, 1938, Dott. G. Poggi-Longostrevi, 'Relation sur la Question des 'Excitants'", ID Chemise: 204766 CIO COMMI-ADMIS 1935 a 1967, IOC Archives.
84. IOC Archive File: ID Chemise: 204766 CIO COMMI-ADMIS 1935 a 1967, IOC Archive.
85. Avery Brundage, Hand written note (undated, likely 1937), Box 77, Folder 'IOC Meeting Minutes', Brundage Archives.

86. Olympic Charter, 1946, International Olympic Committee, "Olympic Rules 1946," 28, IOC Archives.
87. Hunt, *Drug Games*.
88. Ibid.

References

Bahrke, Michael S., and Charles E. Yesalis. *Performance-Enhancing Substances in Sport and Exercise*. Champaign, IL: Human Kinetics, 2002.

Barney, Robert K., Stephen R. Wenn, and Scott G. Martyn. *Selling the Five Rings: The International Olympic Committee and the Rise of Olympic Commercialism*. Salt Lake City: University of Utah Press, 2002.

Davenport-Hines, R. P. T. *The Pursuit of Oblivion: A Global History of Narcotics*. 1st American ed. New York, NY: Norton, 2002.

Dimeo, Paul. *A History of Drug Use in Sport 1876–1976: Beyond Good and Evil*. London: Routledge, 2007.

Dyreson, Mark. *Making the American Team: Sport, Culture, and the Olympic Experience* (Sport and Society). Urbana: University of Illinois Press, 1998.

Findling, John E., and Kimberly D. Pelle. *Encyclopedia of the Modern Olympic Movement*. Westport, CT: Greenwood Press, 2004.

Gleaves, John. "Doped Professionals and Clean Amateurs: Amateurism's Influence on the Modern Philosophy of Anti-Doping." *Journal of Sport History* 38, no. 2 (2011): 401–418.

Gleaves, John. "Enhancing the Odds: Horse Racing, Gambling and the First Anti-Doping Movement in Sport, 1889–1911." *Sport in History* 32, no. 1 (2012): 26–52.

Guttmann, Allen. *From Ritual to Record: The Nature of Modern Sports*. Revised ed. New York, NY: Columbia University Press, 2004.

Hoberman, John. *Mortal Engines: The Science of Performance and the Dehumanization of Sport*. New York, NY: The Free Press, 1992.

Holt, Richard. "The Origins of Amateurism in Victorian Britain, *c*.1850–1890." Paper represented at the North American Society of Sport History Annual Conference, Berkley, CA, June 1–4, 2012.

Hunt, Thomas. *Drug Games: The International Olympic Committee and the Politics of Doping, 1960–2008*. Austin: University of Texas Press, 2011.

Kruger, Arnd. "The Role of Sport in German International Politics, 1918–1945." In *Sport and International Politics: The Impact of Fascism and Communism on Sport*, edited by P. Arnaud and J. Riordan, 79–96. New York, NY: E & FN Spon, 1998.

Llewellyn, Matthew P. "'Viva L'Italia! Viva L'Italia!' Dorando Pietri and the North American Professional Marathon Craze, 1908–1910." *The International Journal of the History of Sport* 25, no. 6 (2008): 710–736.

Llewellyn, Matthew P., and John Gleaves. "The Rise of the Shamateur: The International Olympic Committee and the Preservation of the Amateur Ideal." In *11th International Symposia for Olympic Research: Problems, Possibilities and Promising Practices: Critical Dialogues on the Olympic and Paralympic Games*, edited by International Center for Olympic Studies, 23–28. London: University of Western Ontario, 2012.

Møller, Verner. "Knud Enemark Jensen's Death During the 1960 Rome Olympics: A Search for Truth?" *Sport in History* 25, no. 3 (2005): 452–471.

Muller, Norbert, ed. *Pierre De Coubertin, 1863–1937*. Lausanne: International Olympic Committee, 2000.

Thompson, Chirstopher S. *The Tour de France: A Cultural History*. 2nd ed. Los Angeles: The University of California Press, 2008.

Waddington, Ivan, and Andy Smith. *An Introduction to Drugs in Sport: Addicted to Winning?* London: Routledge, 2009.

A Powerful False Positive: Nationalism, Science and Public Opinion in the 'Oxygen Doping' Allegations Against Japanese Swimmers at the 1932 Olympics

Mark Dyreson and Thomas Rorke

Departments of Kinesiology and History, Pennsylvania State University, USA

At the 1932 Olympic games the Japanese men's swim team upset their heavily favoured American hosts. Among the many explanations offered for the surprising result, some Americans charged that the Japanese team had 'doped' by inhaling supplemental oxygen before they raced. The Japanese admitted to the practice while they and their supporters noted that no rule existed barring such a practice. Nevertheless, allegations flew and attracted the scrutiny of scientists interested in the question of whether or not oxygen enhanced sporting performances. The great majority of commentators concluded that Japan had done nothing illegal or unethical, that Japanese oxygen usage had not given their swimmers any advantage, and that the charges were ultimately a jingoistic attack by certain US swim officials against their rising rival. Nevertheless, the stigma of 'doping' clung to the Japanese team for many decades afterward. Scientists referred to this case in their textbooks, the press regularly re-circulated the charges and IOC officials who began in the 1930s to worry about the use of performance-enhancing substances treated the incident as the first 'evidence' of doping in Olympic history. Nationalism ultimately held more power in shaping the narrative of Japanese 'oxygen doping' than scientific opinion.

'Popeyed Explanations of the Mysterious Marvels from the Orient': The Japan–US Swim Rivalry of the 1930s

In a 1939 article in the *Saturday Evening Post* a US Olympic men's swim coach anticipated a showdown between his swimmers and the mighty Japanese team at the upcoming Tokyo Olympics. Steve Forsyth told one of the magazine's interviewers that the Americans would face a tough battle in Japan. After Japanese swimmers had trounced the US men in 1932 at Los Angeles and then again at 1936 in Berlin, Forsyth admitted that the Japanese had built up an aura of invincibility in Olympic pools that had eroded American confidence and defeated US swimmers psychologically before they had even dipped their toes into the water. Forsyth supported his contention with a vignette from the 1936 Olympics in which a Japanese swimmer used a training swim at Berlin's pool to psych-out his American rivals. Forsyth blustered

> It was the old Japanese hocus-pocus all over again. The awe brought forth by Japan's swimming victories in the 1932 Olympics at Los Angeles has always been a wonder to me. You probably remember the stories about their taking oxygen before the races, and all the

other popeyed explanations of the mysterious marvels from the Orient and their uncanny new stroke.[1]

Six years earlier the claim that Japanese swimmers used oxygen at the 1932 Los Angeles games to spring a surprise upset on what had been since the end of the Great War the world-dominating American swim team was not a 'popeyed explanation' but a white-hot debate in the USA. Charges that the Japanese had illegally 'doped' their swimmers to steal gold medals from Americans flew wildly in the American press. The incident marked the first major scandal in the USA regarding the use of the performance-enhancing substances at the Olympics, setting a pattern for future accusations that the only way foreign athletes could upstage Americans at the games was through the dishonest practice of 'doping'. Curiously, as the scandal played out its substantive elements bubbled into a tempest in a teapot, more of a trifling farce than an international outrage. Still, the Japanese oxygen scandal set a later pattern for condemning foreign Olympians who defeated favoured American champions as drug-gobbling cheats regardless of the validity of the evidence that emerged of their alleged violations of written rules or honorific codes.

The Olympic swimming pool at Los Angeles served as an opening stage for what became a super-charged international rivalry between US and Japanese 'mermen' – as the overwrought American press labelled male swimmers during the era – that would rage until the two nations ceased to engage in proxy aquatic wars and descended into the maelstrom of real and total war in 1941.[2] The Japanese had been sending swimmers to the Olympics since the 1920 games in Antwerp, but until 1932 in Los Angeles Japan's 'mermen' failed to mount a real challenge to US domination of Olympian waters. A few voices in the American press warned US fans that Japan posed a serious challenge in the Olympic pool.[3] Indeed, a Los Angeles psychic predicted a Japanese Olympic victory.[4] Given a decade of utter dominance in Olympic swimming, most of the American public ignored those warnings as if they were all the mumbo–jumbo of carnival seers.[5]

From the other side of the Pacific the Japanese came to Los Angeles brimming with confidence. Japanese journalist Shinichiro Kudo predicted that his nation would finally make a mark in the Olympic pool. 'Though she appears this year as something of a dark horse, tomorrow Nippon will challenge the western world for athletic honors', Kudo predicted.[6] The foreign relations secretary of Japan's national swimming organisation, *Nippon Suizyokyougi Renmei* (the Amateur Swimming Federation of Japan) shared Kudo's sentiments that Japan would challenge the USA for global supremacy in men's swimming. The Japanese official explained that modern 'speed swimming' had only begun in Japan at the turn of the twentieth century but that Japan's aquatic geography, ancient aquatic traditions, and public adoration of water sports had sparked a revolution in Japanese swimming techniques that threatened to upset the established Occidental order in the sport. The Japanese swimming administrator noted that Japan had upset the US team in an international dual meet held in Tokyo in 1931 and would threaten US Olympic hegemony in Los Angeles.[7] An American newspaper, the Los Angeles-based *Rafu Shimpo* that served the Japanese–American community in the US, interviewed Japan's swimmers when they arrived and began to train for the Olympics. 'They were all unanimous in declaring that they would win for Japan', reported *Rafu Shimpo*'s correspondent.[8] None of the Japanese observers who predicted that their nation would challenge the USA in the Olympic pool made any mention of the use of supplemental oxygen as a performance enhancer by Japan's swimmers.

When the USA managed only one gold medal and two bronze medals in the six-event men's swimming programme at Los Angeles while Japan earned five gold medals, four silver medals and two bronze medals, a seismic shock rattled American perceptions of their new swimming rivals. [9]A dazed *New York Times* reporter in a year-end wrap-up of sporting milestones months later admitted that 'Japan quite stole the show'. [10]American writers could indulge in stereotypes about 'brown-skinned seals from the Land of the Cherry Blossoms' but had to reconcile themselves that the major US rival in the Pacific had just shattered American aquatic supremacy.[11]

In the immediate aftermath of the shocking upset, US commentators offered a multitude of explanations for Japan's stunning performances, focusing especially on the scientific and technical wizardry Japanese coaches brought to stroke mechanics. Everyone from the hyperbolic sports columnist Grantland Rice to former American Olympic great and current Hollywood Tarzan Johnny Weissmuller saluted Japan's winners for their application of scientific principles to classic strokes. [12]

The 'Oxygen Doping' Scandal Surfaces

Not a single American observer, however, publicly mentioned the Japanese using oxygen or any form of 'doping' until January of 1933, five months after the Olympic torch had been extinguished in Los Angeles.[13] In a startling allegation reported widely in the press just as a new year began in the Depression-wracked USA, the University of Michigan's renowned aquatics coach Matthew Mann charged that the Japanese had cheated their way to victory. In a searing indictment of Japan, Mann alleged that the Japanese swimmers used an illegal stimulant, proclaimed an American 'war against doping' to counter the nefarious Japanese methods, promised to clean up Olympic pools, and pledged to protect American children against the scourge of illicit substances.[14]

Matthew Mann was an authoritative accuser. A swimming prodigy and national boy champion of England, he immigrated to Canada at the age of 21 and then moved to the USA a year later and became one of his adopted nation's leading coaches. He led various clubs to YMCA and Amateur Athletic Union (AAU) national championships and coached collegiate squads at Syracuse, Harvard, Yale, and the US Naval Academy before settling in for a long stint beginning in 1925 as the coach at Michigan. Mann directed Michigan to a national intercollegiate swimming title in 1927 and then repeated the feat in 1928, 1931, and 1932. In the process Mann earned a reputation as a master of stroke mechanics and as an inspirational leader. An English professor at Michigan who penned the introduction to Mann's text on *Swimming Fundamentals* observed that swimming guru was a 'great genius as a teacher'.[15]

Whether or not Mann was a genius as a teacher, he was certainly an astute provocateur if not overly familiar with the rules regarding 'doping'. The 'illicit' substance Mann accused the Japanese swimmers of ingesting was oxygen, an element not barred during the 1930s by any policy of the IOC or the International Swimming Federation, the governing body for aquatic sports.[16] Not only did sports bureaucracies fail to maintain any policies prohibiting the use of the substance but the question of whether or not oxygen actually enhanced performances in swimming or any other sport was also an open issue in the scientific community in that era, as was the question of whether or not the practice held any potential health risks for imbibing athletes. Indeed, experts at Mann's own University of Michigan raised doubts about the effectiveness of oxygen in boosting performance and cast doubts concerning any dangerous side effects that oxygen usage might create. Dr Frank Lyman, the physician for Michigan's athletic department, observed that the physical effect of inhaling oxygen would last 'only for a breath or two if at all'. Dr Louis H. Newburgh, Professor of Clinical Investigation in Internal Medicine at Michigan's medical school, contended that 'the only effect of oxygen toward greater speed or endurance would be in the minds of the athletes'.[17]

Not only scientists and physicians but other American coaches scoffed at Mann's charges. Robert Kiphuth, Yale's swimming mentor as well as the head coach of the 1932 US Olympic team, immediately dismissed Mann's claims. 'I have found the Japanese to be among the finest sportsmen I have met in my whole experience, and I have absolutely no criticism of their methods of training', Kiphuth proclaimed.[18] Clyde Swendsen, a former Olympic water polo player who coached three Olympic divers who won gold in Los Angeles as well as the lone US men's swimming gold medallist, Clarence 'Buster' Crabbe,[19] sided with Kiphuth. 'Matt Mann's charges that the Japanese doped their swimmers to win the Olympic Games are just poppycock', Swendsen insisted. 'The truth of it is that the Japanese swimmers were just too good and their team organization was almost perfect', Swendsen continued. 'The American Olympic Games swimming team could learn a lot from the Japanese'.[20]

Matt Mann, however, disagreed with his aquatic colleagues. Mann reported that his fellow coaches in the Western Conference (later the Big Ten Conference) were appalled by the Japanese practice and had passed a rule barring the use of oxygen at league meets. Mann announced that he would demand that the National Collegiate Athletic Association (NCAA) adopt an oxygen ban at its next annual meeting. The Michigan coach proclaimed his goal in this crusade was protecting the youth of the USA from what he deemed the clearly unethical and potentially harmful use of oxygen in the quest for faster times in the pool. Mann declared he intended 'to forestall the danger of the practice spreading in this country'.[21]

Mann's Charges Unravel – Contemporary Accounts of the 'Doping' Allegations

Some Olympic observers steered clear of Mann's doping tempest. *Rafu Shimpo*'s correspondents completely ignored the oxygen doping controversy.[22] Other Japanese sources, however, made a spirited defence of their practices. Japanese Olympic leaders freely admitted that they had administered oxygen to their swimmers. Ruyzo Nichimoto, a member of the directorate of the Japanese Aquatic Association, explained that on the advice of Japanese sport medicine experts, team physicians had used oxygen to help their swimmers recover from exhaustion. Nichimoto denied that the inhalations had aided the Japanese athletes in winning any races or that the use of oxygen constituted a form of 'doping'.[23]

Unconvinced by Japanese responses to his accusations Mann pressed his case. The NCAA created a subcommittee to investigate the charges. Ironically, the investigatory committee consisted of just two men, Mann and US Olympic swim coach Kiphuth. The latter aquatic authority vehemently and publicly denied that any 'doping' had taken place.[24]

Mann quickly found himself at odds not only with his fellow American coaches and Japanese swimming authorities but with the American press. William 'Bill' Henry, the sports editor of the *Los Angeles Times* and a major booster of the 1932 Olympics in his hometown, lambasted Mann's 'one man "war against doping"' as 'a little tardy – and a little far-fetched'. Henry pointed out that swimming codes did not bar the practice. He also argued that experts denied that the use of oxygen constituted doping. Henry contended that the 'doctors say it isn't "doping" – as a matter of fact they are agreed that, in the manner in which the Japanese athletes took it in the Olympic Games – it isn't even helpful'. Henry did admit that the practice helped the Japanese upset the US swimmers in Los Angeles but not by giving them an unethical advantage. Instead, in Henry's estimation the use of oxygen represented one component of a masterful training system that kept the Japanese in peak mental and physical condition.[25]

The featured Olympic correspondent for the Associated Press, Alan Gould, took Henry's side in the debate. 'It seems quite all right, in principle, to conduct a "war against doping" in the matter of star swimmers or athletes in general, but it smacks of poor sportsmanship at this date for any American, much less a college coach, to belittle the magnificent victory of Japan's young swimmers in the 1932 Olympics, on the basis that oxygen was used by them as a stimulant or restorative', Gould revealed.

He pointed out that the NCAA had no jurisdiction in the matter anyway and observed that if Mann had any real evidence, then he should take it to the International Swimming Federation, the governing body for Olympic aquatics.[26]

In addition to dismissing Mann's charges, Gould also offered a brief history of doping, which he labelled an 'old story'. Gould pointed out that the use of 'stimulants' by elite athletes was a venerable tradition within the customs and legalities of many sports. 'I have heard it told, seemingly on good evidence, that hypodermic injections were used to sustain some of the competitors in a famous Olympic marathon, also that an over-indulgence of spirits was costly to one of the favorites in his event', Gould continued.[27]

He also recalled that a famous American champion had used sherry and eggnog to win a gold medal.[28] 'Why, therefore, all the clamor, even if the Japanese did use liquid oxygen to stimulate or revive their swimmers?' Gould wondered. 'It was done upon medical advice after a study of the effects', he concluded.[29]

Eleven months later, in late December of 1933, the NCAA convention met at Chicago. In spite of Mann's sensational pledge to go to war on doping and the ensuing storm of controversy that had swirled around the Japanese use of oxygen at the Los Angeles Olympics, the official records of the meeting entirely ignored oxygen, doping, and Japan. The University of Pennsylvania's F.W. Luehring chaired the 'swimming and water sports' committee and penned a report that surveyed twenty years of rule-making in intercollegiate aquatics without a single reference to doping, or to Matt Mann.[30] Robert Kiphuth's name appeared on the list of swimming delegates to the meeting, but Mann's name was nowhere to be found.[31]

A few months later, in April of 1934, Mann effectively gave up his claims about Japanese doping. The April 1934 issue of the *Journal of Health and Physical Education* published an article about the controversy written by Ben Grady, an All-American and NCAA champion in diving at the University of Michigan.[32] The biographical sketch of the author revealed that he was a physical education student at Michigan and that his article had been written under the supervision of Matt Mann. In his study Grady admitted that Japan 'astonished' the world by trouncing the USA at the Los Angeles Olympics and observed that the US defeat had caused enormous consternation and a fervent search for answers. Grady then completely dismissed his mentor's claims that the Japanese had doped their way to an Olympic crown. The Michigan star, under Mann's tutelage, discarded the 'absurd alibi about oxygen by the Japanese swimmers, given wholly to sooth the public's mind'. Through his surrogate Mann apparently admitted that his charges were merely a public relations ploy.[33] In the rest of the article, Grady also discounted theories that the Japanese had invented new and superior swimming strokes. The real answer to Japan's triumph in Los Angeles, according to Grady, was a superior training system and a greater commitment to the discipline required for victory. 'I say', Grady declared

> that the main thing that beat our Olympic team can be summed up in the word *work*. That, and only that, is what beat us and not all this hodge-podge about an entirely different stroke and the use of oxygen.[34]

The Scientists Weigh In

Even as his student admitted that Mann's original doping claims were a smokescreen designed to placate the American public after a startling reversal of US fortunes in the Olympic pool, Mann's charges made oxygen 'doping' a hot topic among sport scientists. Scientific studies of the effects of oxygen on swimmers were conducted not only in Japan but in the USA.[35] Peter V. Karpovich, a leading expert in the field, offered a scientific assessment of the controversy in a 1934 issue of the *Research Quarterly of the American Physical Education Association.*[36] Karpovich was an internationally renowned exercise physiologist and a faculty member at Springfield College, the YMCA training centre in Springfield, Massachusetts. He admitted that Japanese 'doping' controversy at the 1932 Olympics created the impetus for his study. 'The fact that the Japanese Olympic swimming team used oxygen inhalation before the contest and was so victorious aroused general interest in the effects of oxygen breathing upon athletic performance', Karpovich began. 'Could such a procedure affect the speed in swimming?' the Springfield physiologist wondered. 'Some American coaches immediately decided that it could and stated the Japanese swimmers were thereby "doped" and by means of this "unethical" method were able to make such a successful showing', he continued, targeting Mann without naming the Michigan swim leader. 'This question has been presented to the writer on many occasions', Karpovich noted. 'In order to answer this and other concomitant questions the present investigation has been undertaken'.[37]

Karpovich began his investigation with a review of the conflicting scientific literature on the effect of oxygen on athletic performance. He recapped the battle between the eminent early twentieth-century British physiologists Leõnard Hill, Martin Flack, J.F. Mackenzie, C.G. Douglas and J.S. Haldane about whether or not the inhalation of oxygen enhanced the exercise capacity of human populations in general and elite athletes in particular. Karpovich sided with Hill, Flack and Mackenzie in asserting that oxygen enhanced exercise capacity in both athletes and among the general population. [38]

In his experiments to test that hypothesis, he administered oxygen to one group of Springfield's varsity swimmers immediately before they entered the pool and then gave a control group of swimmers oxygen but made them wait several minutes before they raced. His data indicated that the immediate use of oxygen improved performances marginally but that the control group which waited several minutes to swim after they had taken oxygen did not improve at all. In any time period longer than 3 minutes, Karpovich concluded, the benefits of oxygen consumption completely dissipated. 'There is no doubt oxygen taken immediately before strenuous exercise does benefit the person', Karpovich declared. 'It enables him to run or swim faster or perform more work in the same period of time'. However, he dismissed the findings of earlier scientists including Leonard Hill that the impact of oxygen supplements lasted up to 15 minutes. In addition, Karpovich declared that oxygen supplements were completely safe. 'To call oxygen a "dope" is unwarranted', he complained. 'Although it is beyond the scope of a physiological paper to go into a discussion of what is ethical and what is not, nevertheless it might be asked that if the use of sugar is allowed in competition, why should oxygen be excluded?' he queried.

Karpovich then immediately jumped into ethical debate, ignoring the line he had just drawn about the 'scope' of scientific inquiry. Returning to his original concern with assessing whether or not the Japanese had doped in the Los Angeles Olympic pool, Karpovich issued an unqualified endorsement that Japan's victories were absolutely legitimate. 'In view of the fact that the Japanese took oxygen more than five minutes before swimming, it is safe to assume that the oxygen was not responsible in any way for the phenomenal speed', he surmised.[39]

A 1934 issue of the *Journal of the American Medical Association* (*JAMA*) disseminated Karpovich's findings to the nation's physicians and the general public. Not only did the august professional weekly report Karpovich's scientific findings, but it also endorsed his 'ethical' conclusion about Japanese swimmers. 'In the Olympic games held in California in 1932 the Japanese swimming team inhaled oxygen for five minutes about half an hour before competition', *JAMA* noted. 'The charge was made that such inhalations were unethical and that they were largely responsible for the successful showing of the Japanese competitors', the article continued. The *JAMA* essay concluded that Karpovich had provided a definitive answer to the charge, proving that the Japanese swimmers were clean and had won fair and square.[40]

The popular press picked up the story as well but offered even less clarity on the matter. In a series of syndicated columns on the issue, Dr Morris Fishbein came to contradictory conclusions. In a May 1934 opinion, Fishbein ignored Karpovich's study and contended that 'sprint swimmers in recent Olympic games breathed oxygen before entering the races and had a considerable advantage because of that fact', directly contradicting Karpovich's position.[41] In a July 1934 column, Fishbein converted to Karpovich's position, perhaps influenced by the appearance of the *JAMA* report. 'In the Olympic games last year the Japanese swimming team inhaled oxygen just before engaging in competitive performances', Fishbein began. 'At once a great hubbub was raised and charges were made that such a performance was unethical', the syndicated physician observed. 'Now some scientific studies have been made and provide some facts as to just how much the inhaling of oxygen will help the swimmer', Fishbein admitted. Fishbein accurately reported the basic scientific gist of Karpovich's study, that oxygen had no benefit unless swimmers took to the water within 3 minutes of inhalation. However, Fishbein's column did not report the 'ethical' conclusion reached by Karpovich that oxygen did not give Japanese swimmers an edge and that Japan's victories were absolutely clean.[42]

A few months after Fishbein's columns ran in American newspapers, Karpovich decided to take his own views beyond the scientific community and address the general public. In a November 1934 story in *Scholastic*, a weekly magazine that reached many of the nation's secondary school students. Karpovich asserted to the youthful readers that '[v] arious legends have been created in regard to a magical power of oxygen'. He noted the controversy that swirled around the Japanese swimmers' usage of its so-called 'magical powers' at the Los Angeles Olympics and admitted that '[m]any popular magazine and newspapers refer to oxygen as a tonic for athletes that "peps them up"'. Karpovich warned his young readers not to believe what they read in the popular press. 'Unfortunately, these legends, due to their dramatic color, cling to the minds of the people, and it is difficult to dislodge them', he explained. The Springfield College professor then detailed the history of scientific experimentation with oxygen in athletic endeavours, including his own studies of swimmers.[43]

Karpovich observed that thirty years earlier the British research pioneers Leonard Hill, Martin Flack and A.V. Hill had proved that the use of oxygen supplements right before an athletic event significantly increased performance. Karpovich marvelled that Hill had even suggested building a track in a sealed building into which oxygen was pumped in order to lower existing world running records. Karpovich observed that Hill's proposal had scientific merit but was fiscally if not technically impossible to build. Ultimately, the American scholar informed his pupils that he concurred with his famous colleagues that oxygen could improve performance. He observed that his own experiments revealed that taking oxygen right before a short swimming sprint definitely provided a benefit.

However, Karpovich explained, the effect of oxygen only worked its magic when administered within 5 minutes or less of the event. Longer intervals entirely negated the impact of oxygen supplements. 'This should be borne in mind when trying to explain the victory of the Japanese swimmers during the last Olympic games', he warned his many *Scholastic* readers, noting that the much longer intervals between Japanese inhalations and their events completely exonerated them of the 'doping' allegations. 'Some coaches called oxygen a "dope"', Karpovich explained, without mentioning Matt Mann by name in the charge. 'They were wrong', Karpovich declared. 'There is also nothing unethical in the use of oxygen, since it is not a dope', he insisted. In the final analysis the American scientist acquitted the Japanese of all charges that they had 'doped' and concluded that oxygen should be allowed in competition – even if it did not work except when inhaled shortly before events.[44]

Resilient Condemnations Resist Contradictory Evidence

Discredited by scientists, by his fellow Olympic coaches, by leading sportswriters, and even in the pages of one of the nation's most popular school supplements, Mann's original 'doping' charges retained remarkable staying power in American popular imaginations. In a 1935 syndicated column on the possibility of breaking the 4-min barrier in running the mile, a reporter speculated that it might be attainable if a runner donned an oxygen mask. An accompanying cartoon depicted a runner plodding along with a large oxygen tank on his back and a hard-hat diving style contraption on his head. The caption on the drawing read: 'In the last Olympics the Jap swimmers were accused of doping themselves with oxygen. Maybe our 4 min. miler will look like this'.[45] In the accompanying article, the reporter speculating on four-minute miles offered a history of oxygen doping that indicted the Japanese once again for nefarious practices. 'In the last Olympics held at Los Angeles in 1932 the Japanese swimming team which won four races were suspected of resorting to artificial means of doping their swimmers with oxygen in order to win races', the reporter noted, either miscounting the total number of Japanese victories (five) or concluding that one of the gold medals was clean. 'But the records stand and must be accepted as such', he concluded.[46]

In spite of numerous efforts to discredit Mann's assertion that the Japanese 'doped' their way to glory in 1932 Olympics, the Michigan coach's perspective remained a popular if unsubstantiated belief in the popular press. Stories that depicted the Japanese as introducing 'doping' to Olympic sport in 1932 by inhaling oxygen on the deck of the Los Angeles Olympic pool appeared during the 1950s in *Newsweek* and *Sports Illustrated*.[47] In the 1970s the issue of Japanese oxygen 'doping' in 1932 returned to the NCAA convention when Dr Donald Cooper, who served as the chair of the NCAA's Committee on Competitive Safeguards and Medical Aspects of Sport as well as the US Olympic team's head physician, referenced Japanese oxygen usage at the 1932 Olympics in a rambling discourse on drugs in sport. Cooper argued that 'doping' in modern sport 'really got started–so many times in athletics you see people put 2 and 2 together and get 5–in the 1932 Olympics when the Japanese swim team had some great swimmers, but also each time in Los Angeles before they started swimming they were given oxygen'.

Cooper conceded that their 'oxygen doping' had probably not aided the Japanese victories but insisted that Japan had entered a 'grey area' by introducing that practice to the Olympics. 'I might add that, of course, the Japanese had some damned good swimmers there', Cooper observed, while admitting that the scientific data on oxygen and performance did not support the argument that it provided an unfair benefit to imbibers, or, indeed, any benefit at all. Still, Cooper seemed convinced that oxygen had in some unknown way helped the Japanese seize their gold medals from their American rivals. 'There, of course, may be some psychological help', in using oxygen Cooper argued. 'The power of suggestion is fantastic'.[48]

The 'fantastic' power of suggestion certainly influenced scientific assessments of oxygen doping and Japanese scheming, in spite of Karpovich's studies rejecting such allegations. The standard textbook on exercise physiology during the 1930s noted that the use of oxygen at the Olympics by the Japanese had spurred scientific investigation of 'doping'. James McCurdy and Leonard Larson contended that '[r]espiratory efficiency in relation to swimming ability has been a problem for discussion since the 1932 Olympics. It was found that the Japanese swimmers, who were very successful, inhaled oxygen before competition'. The authors cited Karpovich's studies extensively but remained sceptical of his conclusion that oxygen had no substantive ergogenic properties and neglected to mention that the Springfield scientist had exonerated the Japanese of cheating charges.[49]

References to the Japanese instigating the practice of oxygen doping in the Olympics began to appear in exercise science theses and dissertations.[50] In 1968 the kinesiologists Roscoe Conkling Brown and Gerald S. Kenyon included Karpovich's 1934 *Research Quarterly* study in their section on 'Ergogenic Aids' in *Classical Studies on Physical Activity*, observing in their introduction that Japanese deployment of oxygen in Los Angeles had instigated scientific interest in performance enhancement.[51] Many other scientific texts that followed concurred, placing Japanese oxygen inhalation at the 1932 Olympics at ground zero of modern concern with 'doping' in international sport, even as they followed Karpovich and discounted the impact of oxygen on athletic performance.[52]

Japanese 'oxygen doping' also appeared at ground zero of IOC concerns with the spectre of scientific performance enhancement. Within the guarded chambers of the IOC as concern at the highest levels developed during the 1930s that 'deadly stimulants' would wreak havoc on Olympic sport, the phantasm of Japanese 'oxygen doping' became the mythological starting point for IOC examinations of an impending chemically enhanced cheating epidemic. As historians John Gleaves and Matthew Llewellyn have revealed in their excavation of IOC archives regarding the earliest concerns about doping, the very first reports gathered by the Olympic officials in the 1930s referred to just one specific instance of 'doping' practice in Olympic competition – the use of oxygen by Japanese swimmers at Los Angeles.[53]

The impression that the Japanese had 'doped' at the 1932 Olympics maintained remarkable staying power even as the scientific community built a consensus that oxygen had little use as an ergogenic agent in Olympic sports. The evidence condemning the Japanese evaporated while the patina of immorality left by Mann's unsubstantiated charges remained. The desire to cultivate national identities through Olympic sport rather than any consensus on 'oxygen doping' ultimately drove both popular and scientific interest and impressions of Japan's Olympic breakthrough in Los Angeles.

Swimming, Oxygen, and National Identities

An intense swimming rivalry raged between Japan and the USA for the rest of the decade. When R.J. Kiphuth, the coach at Yale who helmed US Olympic swim teams throughout the 1930s, surveyed the rivalry in May of 1934, he offered several reasons for Japan's eclipse of the USA in international men's aquatics. 'Some experts feel that it was due, in large part, to a change in swimming stroke', Kiphuth noted. 'Others feel that it was to due to a manner of living, emphasizing especially the difference in diet', he continued. 'Still others feel that it is due in large part to the psychological attitude, to a willingness to make a greater sacrifice for cause and country', the US Olympic leader contended. Kiphuth concluded that each of those three elements has some merit. He asserted that the most important factor, however, was the creation of a Japanese Swimming Federation that appeared in the wake of Japan's natatorial failures at the 1924 Paris Olympics. Kiphuth explained that this energetic agency had freed Japanese swimming from the bureaucratic sprawl of the Japanese Athletic Association, a conglomerate much like the AAU that controlled US Olympic sports in that era. The emergence of an administrative unit focused solely on swimming had spurred Japan to the top of the global aquatic rankings Kiphuth insisted in a not so veiled criticism of the AAU. Notably absent from Kiphuth's explanations were charges of oxygen doping.[54]

Kiphuth underscored that the swimming rivalry between the USA and Japan was 'friendly, but real'. He cheered the rise of international match meets between the two nations that had taken off following the Los Angeles Olympics, and he looked forward to the 1936 Olympics in Berlin when the American team would have a chance to regain their global crown.[55]

The American team, led by Kiphuth, failed to regain their laurels at the 1936 Olympics. Japan bested the American 'mermen' in Berlin's Olympic pool while in a series of international spectaculars in both nations the quest for victory swung back and forth throughout the 1930s. Claims of 'doping' dropped out of American interpretations of why Japan sustained its swimming dynasty, replaced by a variety of other sweeping assertions. Following Kiphuth's lead some thought the Japanese had invented new strokes in several events that only they could master. Others pointed to the fact that swimming had become a major spectator sport in Japan that drew tens of thousands to meets and put vast resources at their disposal that their US rivals could not match. Some pointed to Japanese militarism and totalitarianism as the cause, arguing that free societies could not compete with the rigid training regimens employed in a nation that submerged individualism into relentless collectivism. Others explained that while US Olympic swimming struggled for attention within the horde of recreations overseen by the AAU, the Japanese had created a stand-alone association devoted solely to aquatic sports that gave them a huge technocratic advantage.[56] Most of these explanations of US failure to retake global swimming dominion from Japan revealed that Americans remained suspicious about Japanese methodologies and critical that Japanese customs somehow corrupted the purer motives that allegedly animated American devotion to sport.

Even Mann himself moved from 'doping' to some of these other explanations. In his 1940 treatise on *Swimming Fundamentals*, the Michigan coach offered a different version of Japanese prowess at the Los Angeles games. 'In the Olympic games of 1932 the swimmers from Japan won all but one of the swimming races, for the Japanese had become seriously interested in swimming in 1928 and had devotedly studied the technique of the champions, using every available mechanical device for recording and analysis, especially very slow motion pictures', Mann speculated.

'They then adopted certain modifications of the American crawl which permitted greater relaxation and in 1932 demonstrated the soundness of their results by winning practically all the races', he concluded.[57]

Mann's alternative account dropped 'doping' but still carried powerful undertones that raised doubts about Japanese motives and behaviours. In a sophisticated variant of an old Western interpretation of Japan, Mann labelled the Japanese clever copycats who built their swimming empire on an American foundation. Apparently Mann was no longer willing to explain away Japanese swimming prowess as the product of doping. Instead, he made them into sly, totalitarian imitators.

In the late 1930s, stories about Japanese oxygen doping still appeared in the American press, but no longer in conjunction with swimming. Instead, Associated Press reports from the front lines of the invasion of China described a Japanese war machine fuelled by performance-enhancing drugs. 'The scientific attention to human energy is one of the ultra-modern touches disclosed in a first-hand inspection of the organization and methods of a Japanese army in the field', reported American war correspondent Elmer Petersen embedded with Japan's military. 'Energy tablets' and oxygen inhalers, Petersen breathlessly reported, were transforming Japanese men into super-soldiers.[58]

Lessons from an Early Olympic Doping Scandal

Soon after Petersen's report, the anticipated renewal of the USA versus Japan rivalry in swimming slated for the 1940 Tokyo Olympics dissolved into the maelstrom of the Second World War. Shortly afterward, Americans faced Japanese not in Olympic pools but on the battlegrounds of the Pacific Theatre. The hyper-national swimming competition between the two nations looked from that later vantage like a prelude to a much bloodier conflict. The animosity and suspicion that produced Matt Mann's dramatic doping charges in 1932 appeared to have reached their inevitable climax as Japan and the USA descended into total war.[59]

In the decades after Japan's cataclysmic defeat in that conflict, nationalism continues to suffuse memories of the 1932 oxygen doping tempest. In Japanese national memories of their feats in Los Angeles in the aftermath of the Second World War, the oxygen doping scandal did not register. Instead, the Japanese fondly recalled a golden moment in their national narrative that floated in a sanitised space disconnected from the harsher realities of Japanese history in the middle of the twentieth century.[60] In the USA in scientific journals and popular recounting, the patina of scandal remained firmly attached to Japan's swimmers even after a mountain of evidence exonerating the Japanese of doping had appeared.

This first major doping scandal in Olympic history underscores the reality that nationalism has historically suffused perceptions of performance-enhancing substances in elite competition. Many of the later doping scandals in Olympic history would become inextricably entwined with the quest for national supremacy through sport.[61] Doping was not ultimately about idealistic concepts such as fair play or even the individual quest for athletic excellence but about national identity and medal counts. The Japanese triumphs stunned American officials and athletes, media and fans, sending them on a quest to explain this unexpected result. Americans manifested an unshakeable certitude that Japan could not possibly have triumphed by adhering to the true spirit of the sport, and cast about for alternative explanations. Those nationalistic lenses account for the remarkable durability of the Japanese 'oxygen doping' narrative long after a variety of experts had discounted those assertions. The alternative American explanations reveal a similar myopia even as they discounted the doping charges. Whether crediting the state support of swimming granted by Japan's totalitarian government, the grinding work ethic of Japanese swimming automatons or the clever emulation of American-invented strokes and methods, they implied that Japanese gold medals in Olympic swimming during the 1930s derived from nebulously nefarious tactics that were ultimately beneath their American rivals. Nationalism drove the discourses about how and why Japan turned the tables on the USA in Olympic pools.

The Japanese oxygen scandal also served as a harbinger for future doping crises. Thin evidence, disputable scientific findings, and complex ethical questions proved no match for partisan rushes to judgement. In this particular case, once many of the facts emerged, it seemed clear that no doping had actually taken place. Once the charges flew, however, they took on a life of their own. A series of scientific experiments, reasoned newspaper columns, and forceful disputations from coaches disputed the sensational claims, but once the accusations were uttered, the assertions that Japan cheated proved impossible to erase from the early folklore of doping.

The first major doping scandal in Olympic history was a false positive but also a result that revealed how doping cases would in the future become dramatic battles over national honour. Playing the drug-cheat card when Americans lose Olympic events that they expect to win remains a classic strategy in expressions of American Olympic nationalism, regardless in many cases of the quality of the evidence. Certainly the USA does not hold exclusive rights to that strategy as other nations have also made widespread use of it. As for the 1932 Japanese Olympic men's swimming team, suspicions of their guilt as the original Olympic 'dopers' retained an amazing power long after the science of ergogenics exonerated their actions. In a contemporary era where rabid denials of doping guilt have far too often been mere smokescreens to protect the reputations of athletes who gluttonously ingested performance enhancers in the quest for Olympic glory, the case of Japan's swimmers in Los Angeles serves as potent reminder that not every allegation is entirely accurate, though precisely what the Japanese athletes and officials believed about their practices remains mysterious. At least the historical record should reveal that while the Japanese utilisation of oxygen marks the rise of widespread scientific and public concern with 'doping', it does not represent the first use of 'dope', or, at least, effective 'dope' in an Olympic venue.

Notes on Contributors

Mark Dyreson is a professor of kinesiology and history at Pennsylvania State University. He is an academic editor for the *International Journal of Sport History*, the co-editor of the Sport in Global Society: Historical Perspectives book series for Routledge Press, and has published several essays and books on the history of modern sport.

Thomas Rorke is a doctoral student in the History and Philosophy of sport programme in the Department of Kinesiology at the Pennsylvania State University. He has researched extensively on the dynamics of national identity formation in international sport.

Notes

1. Steve Forsyth, as told to Phil R. Sheridan, "We Haven't Begun to Swim" *Saturday Evening Post*, July 22, 1939, 20.
2. For a deeper reading of this swimming 'war' see Dyreson, "Imperial 'Deep Play'."
3. "Japanese Confident of Swim Victories," *Los Angeles Times*, June 18, 1932; "'Who's Afraid?' Say Japanese," *Los Angeles Times*, July 7, 1932; "America's Swimming Hopes Invade Cincinnati," *Los Angeles Times*, July 7, 1932; Paul Lowry, "Pick Your Own Champ," *Los Angeles Times*, July 24, 1932; "Swimmers: Here Are Lads You Must Beat," *Los Angeles Times*, July 29, 1932; and Ralph Huston, "Can Reigning Kings Hold Olympic Crowns Great Sport Query," *Los Angeles Times*, July 30, 1932.
4. Mrs Eileen Garrett, visiting Cal Tech under the auspices of the American Institute of Psychical Research, admitted, 'I don't know enough about athletics to predict the points' but cautioned that in her visions: 'I see the Japanese flag flying at the top; underneath that the flag of the United States; third the flag of Germany'. Mrs Garrett's prediction was for not only swimming but the overall medal count in all sports. "Seer Picks Japanese to Win," *Los Angeles Times*, July 12, 1932.

5. Runar Ohls, "Who's Going to Win in the Olympic Games?" *Game & Gossip*, July 1932, 7–8, 60–62 and "N.Y.A.C. Swimmers in the Olympics," *Winged Foot*, August 1932, 19.
6. Shinichiro Kudo, with Leslie LeCron, "Japan Makes Her Bid," *Game & Gossip*, August 1932, 48.
7. Abe, "Swimming Japan," 20–22.
8. "Japanese Olympic Teams Welcomed," *Rafu Shimpo*, July 10, 1932.
9. Yoshnori Suzuki, "Japan's Record in Olympiad History of Modern Sports in Japan," *Japan Magazine,* February 1938, 38–44; Guttmann and Thompson, *Japanese Sports*, 122–125; Allison Danzig, "Japan's Natators Impress Observers," *New York Times*, August 8, 1932; "Japanese Triumph in Olympic Swim; Shatter Meet Record in Taking 800-Meter Relay Test as 10,000 Look On," *New York Times*, August 10, 1932; "Japan's Hatators Provided Feature; Victories in Five of Six Racing Events Were Turned in Chiefly by Youngsters,"*New York Times*, August 15, 1932; Bob Ray, "Crabbe Annexes Swim Thriller by Inches," *Los Angeles Times*, August 11, 1932; Bob Ray, "Japanese Take Honors in Swimming Events," *Los Angeles Times*, August 7, 1932; "Japan's Natators Provided Feature; Victories in Five of Six Racing Events Were Turned in Chiefly by Youngsters," *New York Times*, August 15, 1932; "The Talk of the Town," *New Yorker*, August 20, 1932, 34; and Richard Ely Danielson, "The Olympic Games: Latest Show on Earth as One Man Saw It," *Sportsman,* September 1932, 19–23, 45–46.
10. "Japan's Swimmers Shone in Olympics; Dominated Men's Competition – American Girls Again Were Supreme" *New York Times*, December 25, 1932.
11. "America's Olympic Victory: Athletes of the N.Y.A.C. Do Their Share in Scoring Points; Sexton and Anderson Two Record Breakers With Shot and Discus" *Winged Foot*, September 1932, 7–10. Over the past few decades a burgeoning literature has emerged that more fully places the 1932 Los Angeles Olympics into political, social, and cultural as well as sporting contexts. See, for instance, Dinces, "Padres on Mount Olympus"; Dyreson, "Endless Olympic Bid"; Dyreson, "Johnny Weissmuller and the Old Global Capitalism"; Dyreson, "Marketing National Identity"; Dyreson, "Marketing Weissmuller to the World"; Dyreson, "Republic of Consumption"; Dyreson and Llewellyn, "Los Angeles Is *the* Olympic City"; Keys, *Globalizing Sport*; Keys, "Spreading Peace, Democracy, and Coca Cola®"; Riess, "Power Without Authority"; Welky,"U.S. Journalism and the 1932 Olympics"; White, "Los Angeles Way of Doing Things"; and Yamamoto, "Cheers for Japanese Athletes."
12. Grantland Rice, "Engineers Won for Japanese," *Los Angeles Times*, August 21, 1932 and Bob Ray, "Weissmuller Explains Japanese Success in Olympics," *Los Angeles Times*, August 21, 1932.
13. This claim is based on an exhaustive search of hundreds of major newspapers and dozens of magazines in the USA for any mention of oxygen related to swimming at the 1932 games in both microfilm sources and electronic databases.
14. "Doping of Amateur Athletes Is Charged," *Port Arthur (Texas) News*, January 13, 1933; "Says Japs Doped Swimmers," *Massillon (Ohio) Evening Independent*, January 13, 1933; "Charges Japanese 'Doped' Swimmers," *New York Times*, January 14, 1933.
15. Charles Fries, "'Matt Mann'–Teacher and Coach," in Mann, *Swimming Fundamentals*, viii. Michigan would go on to win future titles under Mann, including eight in a row in 1934, 1935, 1936, 1937, 1938, 1939, 1940 and 1941; and a final title in 1948. In addition to *Swimming Fundamentals*, see 'Matt Mann' of the International Swimming Hall of Fame website http://www.ishof.org/Honorees/65/65mmann.html, accessed May 8, 2013; "Matt Mann" at Wikipedia; *http://en.wikipedia.org/wiki/Matthew_Mann*, accessed May 8, 2013.
16. Gleaves, "Enhancing the Odds" and Gleaves, "Doped Professionals and Clean Amateurs."
17. Newburgh added a warning that administering oxygen 'would do no good and might harm the athlete'. "Says Japs Doped Swimmers," *Massillon (Ohio) Evening Independent*, January 13, 1933 and "Charges Japanese 'Doped' Swimmers," *New York Times*, January 14, 1933.
18. "No Criticism from Kiphuth," *New York Times*, January 14, 1933 and "Yank Swim Coach Scoffs at Jap Doping Charges," *Los Angeles Times*, January 14, 1933.
19. "Clyde Swendsen," International Swimming Hall of Fame website, http://www.ishof.org/Honorees/91/91cswendsen.html, accessed May 9, 2013.
20. "Swendsen Says Japanese Swimmers Just Too Good," *Los Angeles Times*, January 14, 1933.
21. "Charges Japanese 'Doped' Swimmers," *New York Times*, January 14, 1933 and "Doping of Amateur Athletes Is Charged," *Port Arthur (Texas) News*, January 13, 1933.
22. A search of the 1933 editions of *Rafu Shimpo* failed to turn up a single reference to the burgeoning international scandal.

23. "Physicians Advised Oxygen Administered," *Los Angeles Times*, January 14, 1933 and "Japanese Gives Views," *New York Times*, January 14, 1933.
24. "Yank Swim Coach Scoffs at Jap Doping Charges," *Los Angeles Times*, January 14, 1933; "Says Japs Doped Swimmers," *Massillon (Ohio) Evening Independent*, January 13, 1933"; "No Criticism from Kiphuth," *New York Times*, January 14, 1933"; "Charges Japanese 'Doped' Swimmers," *New York Times*, January 14, 1933; and "Doping of Amateur Athletes Is Charged," *Port Arthur (Texas) News*, January 13, 1933.
25. "Bill Henry Says," *Los Angeles Times*, January 14, 1933.
26. Alan Gould, "Sport Slants," *Lawrence (Kansas) Daily Journal-World*, January 23, 1933 and Alan Gould, "Sport Slant," *Moberly (Missouri) Monitor-Index and Democrat*, January 25, 1933.
27. Alan Gould, "Sport Slants," *Lawrence (Kansas) Daily Journal-World*, January 23, 1933 and Alan Gould, "Sport Slant," *Moberly (Missouri) Monitor-Index and Democrat*, January 25, 1933.
28. Though he does not include strychnine in the list of the 'doping' cocktail, Gould seems to be referring to the medicinal slurry administered to marathon champion Thomas Hicks by the physician Charles Lucas during the 1904 St Louis Olympics. In 1905 Lucas published an extensive account of his experiments on Hicks in *The Olympic Games*.
29. Alan Gould, "Sport Slants," *Lawrence (Kansas) Daily Journal-World*, January 23, 1933 and Alan Gould, "Sport Slant," *Moberly (Missouri) Monitor-Index and Democrat*, January 25, 1933.
30. Luehring, "Swimming and Water Sports," in *Proceedings of the Twenty-Eighth Annual Convention*. Luehring indicates a detailed report of all the committee's work appears in the September 1933 issue of the *NCAA Bulletin*, which we have been unable to obtain.
31. "Roll of Members," 6–13, and "Delegates and Visitors Present," pp. 14–16, in *Proceedings of the Twenty-Eighth Annual Convention*.
32. Grady, "Americans, Japanese, and Swimming," 35, 58. Grady tried out for but failed to make the 1936 US Olympic team in springboard diving. http://www.usaswimming.org/_Rainbow/Documents/cd7383ce-cdf5-48eb-812a-06d8a435497c/1936TrialsResults.pdf, accessed October 25, 2013. Grady went on to a long career as a swimming coach at the University of Pittsburgh and, like his mentor Mann, became a prominent author of texts on aquatic sports. "Ben Grady Wins Award," *Pittsburgh Post-Gazette*, March 27, 1964 and Barr, Grady, and Higgins, *Swimming and Diving*.
33. Grady, "Americans, Japanese, and Swimming," 35.
34. Ibid., 58.
35. On the Japanese side see Teruoka, "Die Ama und ihre Arbeit."
36. For biographical data on Karpovich see Todd and Todd, "Peter V. Karpovich." In the 1954 Karpovich served as one of the founders of the American College of Sports Medicine. Berryman, *Out of Many, One*.
37. Karpovich, "Effect of Oxygen Inhalation," 24–30.
38. Ibid.
39. Ibid.
40. "Oxygen Inhalation and Athletic Activity," 32.
41. Dr Morris Fishbein, "You Can't Live Five Minutes without Oxygen," *Billings (Montana) Gazette*, May 18, 1934.
42. Dr Morris Fishbein, "Oxygen Aids Athletes Just Before Events," *Billings (Montana) Gazette*, July 7, 1934 and Dr Morris Fishbein, "Oxygen Aids Athletes Just Before Events," *Coshocton (Wisconsin) Tribune*, July 13, 1934.
43. Peter V. Karpovich, "Oxygen Tests on Athletes," *Scholastic*, November 24, 1934, 28.
44. Karpovich, "Oxygen Tests on Athletes," 28. For additional evidence of Hill and Flack's support of oxygen usage in sport see "To Oxygenize Athletes: Plan of Prof. Leonard Hill, F.R.S., to Break All World's Sporting Records," *New York Times*, August 23, 1908.
45. John J. Romano, "Ferris Predicts 4-Minute Mile; Bonthron Says 'Impossible,'" *Butte Montana Standard*, February 17, 1935. Lest the image of a runner in with an oxygen mask and tank seem too whimsical to have ever been seriously considered, according to *Scientific American* in 1912 the eminent British scientist, Sir Edwin Ray Lankester, the evolutionary biologist who directed the natural history exhibits at the British Museum, petitioned the organisers of the Stockholm Olympics to permit a runner under his guidance to compete in the marathon while using a supplemental oxygen tank. The editors of the influential US journal condemned Lankester's effort as an affront to sportsmanship and labelled it as 'doping'. "Doping Athletes with Oxygen," *Scientific American*, April 6, 1912, 302.

46. Fishbein, "Oxygen Aids Athletes Just Before Events."
47. "Have a Whiff," *Newsweek*, December 15, 1952, 91; "Philadelphia Heirlooms, Fame & Fortune on Horseback, Are Pep-up Pills Cricket?" *Sports Illustrated*, November 15, 1954, 20.
48. *Proceedings of the 65th Annual Convention*, 69.
49. McCurdy and Larson, *Physiology of Exercise*, 248.
50. Mary Margaret Yost, "The Effect of 100 Per Cent Oxygen Inhalation on Performance and Recovery in Swimming," Ph.D. thesis, Ohio State University, 1949; Michael D. Giese, "The Effects of 100 Percent Oxygen Inhalation during Recovery in Intermittent Work," M.S. thesis, University of Wisconsin–Madison, 1972.
51. They accurately noted in their introduction that Karpovich's study cleared the Japanese of doping. Brown and Kenyon, *Classical Studies on Physical Activity*, 390–395.
52. Morgan and Corbin, *Ergogenic Aids and Muscular Performance*, 325; Klafs and Arnheim, *Modern Principles of Athletic Training*, 142; Wagenvoord, *Swim Book*, 13; Jenkins, *Sports Science Handbook*, Volume 2: I–Z, 158; and Kenney, Wilmore, and Costill, *Physiology of Sport and Exercise*, 414.
53. Gleaves and Lewellyn cite a 1938 report to the IOC by an Italian doctor, G. Poggi-Longostrevi, "Relation sur la Question des 'Excitants'", held in the IOC archives in Lausanne, Switzerland. Gleaves and Llewellyn, "Sport, Drugs, and Amateurism."
54. Kiphuth, "Japan Challenges America in the Water," *Literary Digest*, May 12, 1934, 24.
55. Ibid.
56. Kiphuth, "Japan Challenges America," 24; Lawson Robertson, "Rising Sons: Japan's Bid for Athletic Supremacy," *Saturday Evening Post*, June 23, 1935, 10–11, 67–68; Forsyth, "We Haven't Begun to Swim," *Saturday Evening Post*, July 22, 1939, 20–21, 33–36.
57. Mann, *Swimming Fundamentals*, 101.
58. Elmer Peterson, "'Energy Tablets' Spur on Japan's Weary Soldiers," *Chicago Tribune*, May 24, 1938 and "Japanese Soldiers Take 'Energy Tablets,' Inhale Oxygen to Obtain New Strength," *New York Times*, May 24, 1938.
59. The same racial and national ideologies that drove the oxygen doping controversy contributed to the war. Historians have long identified racial and national ideologies as central factors in both the origin and savagery of the Pacific War. Dover, *War without Mercy*; Iriye, *Origins of the Second World War*; Thompson, *Empires of the Pacific*.
60. The reminiscence of one of the Japanese gold medallists, Masaji Kiyokawa, illuminates this disconnection. Kiyokawa, "My Golden Moment," 10–14. See also, Neihaus, "Swimming into Memory," 430–443.
61. Hunt, *Drug Games*.

References

Abe, K. "Swimming Japan: What Can it Do in the Coming Olympiad?" *Journal of Health and Physical* 3, no. 6 (1932): 20–22.

Barr, Alfred, Ben Grady, and John Higgins. "Swimming and Diving." Annapolis, MD: United States Naval Institute, 1954.

Berryman, Jack W. *Out of Many, One: A History of the American College of Sports Medicine*. Champaign, IL: Human Kinetics, 1995.

Brown, Roscoe Conkling, and Gerald S. Kenyon, eds. *Classical Studies on Physical Activity*. Englewood Cliffs, NJ: Prentice-Hall, 1968.

Dinces, Sean. "Padres on Mount Olympus: Los Angeles and the Production of the 1932 Olympic Mega-Event." *Journal of Sport History* 32, no. 2 (2005): 137–166.

Dover, John W. *War Without Mercy: Race and Power in the Pacific War*. New York: Pantheon Books, 1986.

Dyreson, Mark. "Marketing National Identity: The Olympic Games of 1932 and American Culture." *Olympika: The International Journal of Olympic Studies* 4 (1995): 23–48.

Dyreson, Mark. "The Endless Olympic Bid: Los Angeles and the Advertisement of the American West." *Journal of the West* 47, no. 4 (2008): 26–39.

Dyreson, Mark. "Johnny Weissmuller and the Old Global Capitalism: The Origins of the Federal Blueprint for Selling American Culture to the World." *International Journal of the History of Sport* 25, no. 2 (2008): 268–283.

Dyreson, Mark. "Marketing Weissmuller to the World: Hollywood's Olympics and Federal Schemes for Americanization Through Sport." *International Journal of the History of Sport* 25, no. 2 (2008): 284–306.
Dyreson, Mark. "Imperial 'Deep Play': Reading Sport and Visions of the Five Empires of the 'New World': 1919–1941." *International Journal of the History of Sport* 28, no. 17 (2011): 2415–2441.
Dyreson, Mark. "The Republic of Consumption at the Olympic Games: Globalization, Americanization, and Californization." *Journal of Global History* 8, no. 2 (2013): 256–278.
Dyreson, Mark, and Matthew Llewellyn. "Los Angeles Is *the* Olympic City: Legacies of 1932 and 1984." *International Journal of the History of Sport* 25, no. 14 (2008): 1991–2018.
Gleaves, John. "Doped Professionals and Clean Amateurs: Amateurism's Influence on the Modern Anti-Doping Movement." *Journal of Sport History* 38, no. 2 (2011): 401–418.
Gleaves, John. "Enhancing the Odds: Horse Racing, Gambling and the First Anti-Doping Movement in Sport, 1889–1911." *Sport in History* 32, no. 1 (2012): 26–52.
Gleaves, John, and Matthew Llewellyn. "Sport, Drugs, and Amateurism: Tracing the Cultural Origins of Anti-Doping Rules in International Sport." *International Journal of the History of Sport* 31, no. 5 (2014).
Grady, Ben. "Americans, Japanese, and Swimming." *Journal of Health and Physical Education* 5 (1934): 35–58.
Guttmann, Allen, and Lee Thompson. *Japanese Sports: A History*. Honolulu: University of Hawai'i Press, 2001.
Hunt, Thomas. *Drug Games: The International Olympic Committee and the Politics of Doping, 1960–2008*. Austin, TX: University of Texas Press, 2010.
Iriye, Akira. *The Origins of the Second World War in Asia and the Pacific*. New York: Longman, 1987.
Jenkins, Simon P. R. *Sports Science Handbook: The Essential Guide to Kinesiology, Sport and Exercise Science*, Volume 2: I–Z. Brentwood: Multi-Science, 2005.
Karpovich, Peter V. "The Effect of Oxygen Inhalation on Swimming Performance." *Research Quarterly of the American Physical Education Association* 5, no. 2 (1934): 24–30.
Kenney, W. Larry, Jack H. Wilmore, and David L. Costill. *Physiology of Sport and Exercise*, 5th ed. Champaign, IL: Human Kinetics, 2012.
Keys, Barbara. "Spreading Peace, Democracy, and Coca Cola®: Sport and American Cultural Expansion in the 1930s." *Diplomatic History* 28 (2004): 165–196.
Keys, Barbara. *Globalizing Sport: National Rivalry and International Community in the 1930s*. Cambridge: Harvard University Press, 2006.
Kiyokawa, Masaji. "My Golden Moment: Swimming into Olympic History." *Journal of Olympic History* 5, no. 3 (1997): 10–14.
Klafs, Carl E., and Daniel D. Arnheim. *Modern Principles of Athletic Training: The Science of Sports Injury Prevention and Management*., 4th ed. St. Louis, MO: Mosby, 1977.
Lucas, Charles J. P. *The Olympic Games: 1904*. St Louis, MO: Woodward & Tiernan, 1905.
Mann, Matt. *Swimming Fundamentals*. New York: Prentice Hall, 1940.
McCurdy, James Huff, and Leonard A. Larson. *The Physiology of Exercise: A Text-Book for Students of Physical Education*. Philadelphia, PA: Lea & Febiger, 1939.
Morgan, William P., and Charles B. Corbin. *Ergogenic Aids and Muscular Performance*. New York: Academic Press, 1972.
National Collegiate Athletic Association. "Proceedings of the Twenty-Eighth Annual Convention of the National Collegiate Athletic Association.", December 30, 1933, Chicago, IL, 1933.
National Collegiate Athletic Association. *Proceedings of the 65th Annual Convention of the National Collegiate Athletic Association*. Kansas City, MS: NCAA, 1971.
Neihaus, Andreas. "Swimming into Memory: The Los Angeles Olympics (1932) as Japanese *lieu de mémoire*." *Sport in Society: Cultures, Commerce, Media, Politics* 14, no. 4 (2011): 430–443.
"Oxygen Inhalation and Athletic Activity." *Journal of the American Medical Association* 103, no. 7 (1934): 32.
Riess, Steve. "Power Without Authority: Los Angeles' Elites and the Construction of the Coliseum." *Journal of Sport History* 8, no. 1 (1981): 50–65.
Teruoka, Gito. "Die Ama und ihre Arbeit." *Arbeitsphysiologie* 5, no. 3 (1932): 239–251.
Thompson, Robert Smith. *Empires on the Pacific: World War II and the Struggle for the Mastery of Asia*. New York: Basic Books, 2001.

Todd, Jan, and Terry Todd. "Peter V. Karpovich: Transforming the Strength Paradigm." *Journal of Strength Conditioning Research* 17, no. 2 (2003): 213–220.

Wagenvoord, James. *The Swim Book.* Indianapolis, IN: Bobbs-Merrill, 1980.

Welky, David. "Viking Girls, Mermaids, and Little Brown Men: U.S. Journalism and the 1932 Olympics." *Journal of Sport History* 24, no. 1 (1997): 24–49.

White, Jeremy. "The Los Angeles Way of Doing Things: The Olympic Village and the Practice of Boosterism." *Olympika: The International Journal of Olympic Studies* 11 (2000): 79–116.

Yamamoto, Eriko. "Cheers for Japanese Athletes: The 1932 Los Angeles Olympics and the Japanese American Community." *Pacific Historical Review* 69, no. 3 (2000): 399–429.

The Myth of the Nazi Steroid

Marcel Reinold[a] and John Hoberman[b]

[a]*Institute for Sport and Exercise Sciences, Sport Pedagogy and History, University of Münster, Münster, Germany;* [b]*Department of Germanic Studies, University of Texas, Austin, TX, USA*

The myth of the 'Nazi steroid' has persisted over the past four decades in the absence of any reliable evidence to support it. This essay traces the myth back to a short article that appeared in the respectable American journal *Science*. Our examination of the paper trail suggests that the myth was started by a rumour that the *Science* journalist converted into a hypothesis. Two factors account for the impressive career of this fantasy. First, it is striking how many writers were willing to transmit this claim to their readers in an uncritical manner on the undocumented assumption that it was a plausible idea. The second factor is how the world has imagined the Nazi regime. It has been credited with the capacity to commit virtually any perverse act, no matter how improbable or bizarre it may seem. In the last analysis, the myth of the 'Nazi steroid' confirms once again a widespread fascination with the Nazis that includes a masculine megalomania that is best represented by the legendary sadism of the Nazi criminal regime. It is, therefore, no accident that the 'male hormone' and its reputation as a catalyser of male aggression have become a symbol of the Nazi ethos.

> In the darkest days of World War II, when a secret super-soldier serum transformed 90-pound weakling Steve Rogers into a physically perfect specimen of humanity, a legend was born – Captain America! As the living symbol of his country and the principles it represents, he fought valiantly to help the United States and its allies win that long-ago war ... but his personal war continues to this day. For as long as tyranny and evil exist, Captain America will never pause in his quest to bring liberty and justice to all! (Marvel Masterpieces ad for CAPTAIN AMERICA)

Introduction

Despite 40 years of undocumented reports to the contrary, there are no credible reports of the Nazis' alleged use of anabolic steroids for military purposes.[1] The myth of the Nazi steroid is briefly analysed in John Hoberman's *Mortal Engines: The Science of Performance and the Dehumanization of Sport* (1992). 'Inside the drug-ridden worlds of high-performance sport and bodybuilding', he argues, 'the basic fantasy of Nazi-inspired scientific ingenuity has lived on as the myth of the "Nazi steroid" – a perfect commingling of storm-trooper "masculinity" and the secret science of the East German sports laboratories combined into a single idea. ... Combining Nazis and male hormones fulfills a longstanding stereotype about German national character', in that the Nazis promulgated the most extreme veneration of masculinity in the form of the German male as both warrior and racial paragon.[2] Given that testosterone was not synthesised until 1935, it is not surprising that there is no evidence that anabolic steroids were used at the 1936 Berlin Olympic Games, either; the time factor alone would have ruled out their use by German athletes or anyone else.[3] But inevitably, and notwithstanding the combination of absent evidence and sheer implausibility, the profound appeal of the Nazi-steroid affinity could not leave this stone unturned; Paul Dimeo has thus reported a claim 'that Hitler ensured German athletes had access to doping drugs for the 1936 Olympics in Berlin'.[4]

In this paper, we will critically discuss the myth of the Nazi steroid relating to military and high-performance sports. Before we outline the myth in some detail, we have to address contextual questions regarding what actually constituted doping and anti-doping during the interwar and Nazi era. We will then present a brief overview of research on performance-enhancing substances during this period.

Doping: Contemporary Definition, Regulation and Moral Implications

The meaning of the term 'doping' has varied over time.[5] A historically adequate understanding of the term during the interwar and Nazi periods takes into account that 'doping' primarily referred to stimulants. Stimulants were considered to be the most effective and also the most dangerous performance-enhancing substances in sports. They represented the prototype of doping substances until the 1970s. Used shortly before competitions, they were said to cause temporary performance enhancement that could lead to a dangerous state of exhaustion since they allow athletes to perform beyond their 'normal' or 'natural' physical capacity. The crucial problem, however, is that several other kinds of substances could also be classified as 'abnormal', 'unnatural' or 'harmful'. It is important to note that the concept of doping relies on normative distinctions between allowed and prohibited substances and methods for performance-enhancement. In fact, drawing a clear line between legitimate nutritional supplements and objectionable doping substances constituted a crucial problem. The sources show no consensus on how to classify performance-enhancing drugs and methods that are not stimulants. One controversy during the interwar period was the broadly discussed question of whether the use of ultraviolet rays was to be considered an 'unnatural', 'abnormal' and 'unhealthy' form of physical preparation and thus constituted doping.[6] In contrast, the question of whether the use of testosterone constitutes doping was never discussed during the interwar or Nazi periods. The reason was that it did not play a role in performance-enhancement in sports during this time. This situation fundamentally changed during the 1960s and 1970s, when anabolic steroids became the most important performance-enhancing drugs in sports. However, the question of whether the use of anabolic steroids constituted doping remained unclear. Even as late as 1970, the Austrian sport physician and anti-doping pioneer Ludwig Prokop had to admit that these substances constituted an 'unsolved and ambiguous problem ... which lacks consensus and uniform standards'.[7]

There is another significant difference between doping during the interwar and Nazi periods and doping today. Compared to today's sophisticated anti-doping system with formalised rules, tests and bans, there were hardly any anti-doping measures worldwide during the first half of the twentieth century. In fact, drug testing was limited to equestrian sports.[8] Doping in human sports was neither prosecuted nor sanctioned. Most sports federations had not implemented any kinds of anti-doping rules. In fact, the International Amateur Athletic Federation (IAAF) seems to be the only international federation in human sports, which had implemented an anti-doping rule during the interwar period. Only few German federations had implemented any kind of anti-doping rules.

Furthermore, the significance of these rules should not be overestimated. In comparison to today's Code of the World Anti-Doping Agency, which currently runs to 136 pages, the rules of the German Athletic Federation (Deutsche Sportbehörde für Leichtathletik) of 1927 and the German Amateur Boxing Federation (Deutscher Reichsverband für Amateur-Boxen) of 1929 consisted of just one short sentence.[9] The IAAF anti-doping rule of 1928 defined and banned doping in only a few more sentences. According to this rule:

> Doping is the use of any stimulant not normally employed to increase the power of action in athletic competition above the average. Any person knowingly acting or assisting as explained above shall be excluded from any place where these rules are in force, or, if he as a competitor, be suspended for a time or otherwise, from participating in amateur athletics under the jurisdiction of this federation.[10]

However, neither the rules of the German federations nor the IAAF rule indicated how this moral code might be policed. Practical aspects of anti-doping, such as detection methods and legal proceedings, were not mentioned. We also have no evidence that concrete measures were taken to enforce the rules. In fact, athletes were subjected to experimental drug tests in the 1950s and were sanctioned during the 1960s for the first time.

Furthermore, it is important to note that the IAAF rule explicitly referred to amateur athletics. In fact, doping was banned only in amateur and not in professional sports. For example, in a case of doping where a German sport physician administered drugs to several athletes, the German Association of Sports Physicians clearly rejected drug use in amateur sports in 1927. In professional sports, however, it was emphasised that 'doping ... can easily be justified because the focus doesn't lie on the success in sports but on social success'.[11]

Briefly summarised, by the period when the Nazi steroid use allegedly occurred, doping was somehow morally offensive in amateur sports but rarely prohibited by formalised rules and, above all, neither prosecuted nor sanctioned. Furthermore, it was primarily stimulants used shortly before the competition that were considered as doping at that time. This is very different from what later decades would bring.

Research on Performance-Enhancing Substances

Modern scientific physiology and pharmacology developed in the second half of the nineteenth century. German researchers such as Helmholtz, du Bois-Reymond, Virchov, Buchheim and Schmiedeberg played prominent roles in the development of these sciences.[12] Furthermore, during that period public health became politically relevant in Germany, leading to the first legislative interventions regarding social insurance and hygiene. The 1920s and, especially, the Nazi-period saw the golden age of social as well as racial hygiene.[13] The fact that Germany prepared and fought two world wars significantly accelerated research in the field of public health, hygiene and performance enhancement. It was in military research that experiments on diet and performance-enhancing drugs were carried out to increase military capacity of the Wehrmacht, Luftwaffe and Kriegsmarine.[14]

Nutritional research for military purposes was a new field in Germany and was first conducted in the context of World War I. The Kaiser-Wilhelm-Institute for Occupational Physiology (Kaiser-Wilhelm-Institut für Arbeitsphysiologie) was founded just before the start of World War I and began with nutrition research on behalf of the War Ministry. Nutrition research for military purposes stopped after World War I in the course of disarmament and demobilisation due to the Treaty of Versailles. However, the

Kaiser-Wilhelm-Institute for Occupational Physiology started nutritional and pharmacological research for military purposes again in the mid-1920s and it intensified during the 1930s. In 1937, a more specialised institute for military purposes under the direction of the German Army and called the 'Institute for Occupational and Military Physiology' (Institut für Arbeits- und Wehrphysiologie) was founded and quickly established a close relationship with the German food industry.[15]

Politicians, researchers and German industry pushed nutritional and pharmacological research not only for military use but also for purposes of public health. In 1920, the Emergency Association of German Science (Notgemeinschaft der deutschen Wissenschaft) was founded. This association was the predecessor institution of the German Research Foundation (Deutsche Forschungsgemeinschaft), currently the most important research foundation in Germany. Three characteristics of the Emergency Association of German Science should be highlighted here. First, the institution was established in order to support the inadequate German universities and science in general during the difficult years after World War I. However, as already mentioned, it remained an outstanding institution within the German research landscape. Second, as a state-financed institution, it focused its research on projects that were considered to be politically relevant. Public health became increasingly important during the nineteenth century and developed into an extreme form during the Nazi period. The search for new and effective pharmacological substances, as well as research on effects and applications, fit the political goals of public health and industrial productivity during the Nazi era. Third, close links between the Emergency Association of German Science and the German pharmaceutical industry existed from the beginning. The pharmaceutical industry was well aware of the commercial potential of pharmacological innovations.[16]

To summarise, research projects in the Weimar Republic and especially during the Nazi period in the field of nutrition and pharmacology were closely linked to political objectives, first and foremost public health, increased work capacity and military power, as well as the commercial interests of the developing pharmaceutical industry. The establishment of institutions such as the Kaiser-Wilhelm-Institute for Occupational Physiology, the Institute for Occupational and Military Physiology or the Emergency Association of German Science exemplifies the institutionalised connection between political, commercial and scientific objectives. At a time when public health, industrial productivity and military power became extraordinarily important political goals, and the developing pharmaceutical industry pushed their commercial interests, research on pharmacological substances was no longer just a matter of science but also became politically and economically relevant. In fact, pharmacological research on hormones, vitamins or amphetamines cannot be understood without taking into account the close connections between politics, industry and science.[17]

Vitamins were the primary focus in the 1920s and 1930s, finally leading to industrial mass production during the mid-1930s. Vitamin C became especially popular in the wider society since it was no longer exclusively used to treat diseases like scurvy but was also used preventively and – even more important in the context of doping – for performance enhancement in everyday life. Vitamins were also increasingly used for military purposes. Hofmann-La Roche, the market leader in the production of vitamin C, tripled its production between 1939 and 1943, primarily because of the growing demand from the German army.[18] In fact, German soldiers were supplied with vitamins starting in the winter of 1940. Of the 186,000 kilograms of vitamins that were produced in 1943 by the companies Hofmann-La Roche, Merck and I.G. Farben, 100,000 kilograms were used by the Wehrmacht.[19]

The most famous performance-enhancing substance used by German soldiers was the highly effective amphetamine Pervitin. The Institute for Occupational and Military Physiology, in cooperation with the Kaiser-Wilhelm Institute and the Temmler company, carried out a series of military tests examining Pervitin beginning in 1937. Pervitin was then systematically introduced into the medical practice of the Wehrmacht, Luftwaffe and Kriegsmarine.[20] At first, there were few concerns about potential side effects of the drug.[21] However, this view quickly changed. Leonardo Conti, the leader of the German Medical Association in the Third Reich, stated in 1940:

> Whoever wants to combat fatigue with Pervitin can be sure that the collapse will come sooner or later. It is correct that the drug may be used once by a high-performance fighter pilot who has to fly two hours more. However, it shall not be used to combat fatigue in every situation.[22]

Growing concerns about the potential side effects and addiction were the reasons why Pervitin finally fell under the Opium Act in 1941.[23]

The Myth is Born

In contrast to Pervitin's use by the military, which is well documented, the question of testosterone use for performance-enhancement in the German Army is far more controversial. Testosterone was first synthesised independently by the German Adolf Butenandt and the Croatian Leopold Ruzicka in1935 and manufactured in commercial quantities one year later.[24] Against this background, it seems reasonable to assume that the German Wehrmacht could have used testosterone for military purposes. In fact, a number of writers have made such claims, though under scrutiny none of these claims meet the most basic standards of good historiography.

The Nazi steroid story appears to begin in the auditorium of the Masonic Temple in Detroit at the 1972 Mr America bodybuilding contest. Present at this event was the young science journalist Nicholas Wade, who is now a science writer for the *New York Times*. His report for *Science* magazine, 'Anabolic Steroids: Doctors Denounce Them, But Athletes Aren't Listening', reads well 40 years after it was published. The essay presented a comprehensive survey of contemporary doping practices at a time when doctors routinely debunked steroids as useless for performance-enhancement and pointed to their medical dangers. The seminal moment in the history of the 'Nazi steroid' occurred when the author reports:

> The first use of male steroids to improve performance is said to have been in World War II, when German troops took them before battle to enhance aggressiveness.[25]

This is the earliest claim about the Nazi steroid of which we are aware. In April 2013, the author told us he had been asked about this before and had been unable to find the source of the report. He also pointed out that in his article he had treated it as hearsay evidence.[26] The fact that Wade was mingling with steroid-using bodybuilders may answer the question of how this topic came to his attention, even if we cannot know where the hypothetical informant might have picked up the rumour about the Nazis' military use of anabolic steroids. What we can do is recognise the affinity between the hyper-masculine ideology of this criminal regime and a substance that by 1972 had long been known as 'the male hormone'.[27] What one makes of this affinity is a matter of perspective. For a doctor who administers an anabolic steroid as medical therapy, the association is irrelevant. For some bodybuilders and motorcycle gang members, it will give the drug a special cachet. But for the serious steroid proponent for whom androgenic drugs are a way of life, the myth of the

Nazi steroid can be one more way to defame an entire class of useful drugs. For example, the steroid writer and promoter Millard Baker wrote in 2012:

> What better way to demonize steroids than to link them to evil, Nazi doctors?! Schutz-Staffel soldiers were allegedly injected with steroids to increase their aggressiveness before battle in Adolf Hitler's Nazi Germany. The specter of steroids has been reported as one of the factors underlying the violence and atrocities in Nazi-occupied territories and the systematic state-sponsored murder of millions of Jews during the Holocaust. Anything associated with Nazi Germany has been considered sinister and malicious. Steroids are no exception.[28]

It is worth noting that Baker presents this protest against 'anti-steroid propaganda' – in effect, an alleged Nazi-exploiting smear campaign – in an explicitly philo-Semitic text that sings the praises of Jewish scientists who, according to Baker, contributed to the development of the anabolic steroid. Whereas Dimeo, as well as Rob Beamish and Ian Ritchie[29] seem to disapprove of unwarranted and unflattering associations between steroids and sadistic totalitarians; their disapproval, unlike Baker's, does not take the form of steroid evangelism.

The later influence of Wade's 1972 article cannot be precisely determined. It is cited in 1984 by Haupt and Rovere, who write:

> Anabolic steroids were reportedly first used during World War II when they were given to German troops to enhance their aggressiveness.[30]

Haupt and Rovere are cited in 1989 by Wadler and Hainline, who recite what is by now a familiar line:

> During World War II, German troops employed anabolic steroids in efforts to enhance their muscle strength and increase their aggressiveness.[31]

Wadler and Hainline also cite a 1985 article by Perlmutter and Lowenthal.[32] In 1987 the steroid historian Terry Todd writes:

> There is also evidence that the Germans continued their experimentation during the war, and even administered testosterone to some storm troopers to increase their aggressiveness. Dr. William Taylor has speculated that since Hitler had used the drug, it might have accounted for some of the mood swings and aggressiveness of the German fuhrer [*sic*].[33]

Todd's footnote illustrates how unreliable and/or unverifiable sources can become embedded in a sequence of citations that can be perpetuated indefinitely. In this case, an apparently fictional source (Silverman, 'Guaranteed Aggression') is cited by a source to which we do not have access ('Hitler's Final Days', *American Medical News*), which in turn had been cited by the steroids writer William Taylor, in an unpublished paper presented at a symposium on *Ethical Issues in the Treatment of Children and Athletes with Human Growth Hormone*.[34] Taylor's comments on the Nazis and anabolic steroids appear in print in 1991 in *Macho Medicine: A History of the Anabolic Steroid Epidemic*; what is more, these remarks are both imprecise and somewhat incoherent.[35] As Beamish pointed out, Taylor repeated his claims in the second edition of *Anabolic Steroids and the Athlete* in 2002.[36] Interestingly, in contrast to the second edition, the first edition of Taylor's *Anabolic Steroids and the Athlete* of 1982 did not mention the Nazi steroid myth. Beamish emphasises that this difference has to do with Taylor's underlying intentions. Taylor's agenda in 1982 was to overcome sporting officials' obstruction of further scientific investigation. Taylor argued against demonising anabolic steroids on a non-scientific basis by claiming that 'prescribing steroids to athletes in a controlled fashion with regular physician follow-up visits is less dangerous than prescribing many – if not most – of the medications currently available'.[37] Steroid use, in his view of 1982, should be 'like elective surgery, where there is informed consent following an explanation of the risks'.[38] Therefore, Taylor felt that scientific facts about anabolic steroids were important to provide accurate information to athletes. Taylor's position has changed considerably since the middle of the 1980s. In *Hormonal Manipulation: A New Era of Monstrous Athletes* of 1985, Taylor emphasised the negative side effects and clearly argued against the use of these drugs in sports. His agenda of demonising anabolic steroids continued in *Macho Medicine* of 1991 and the second edition of *Anabolic Steroids and the Athlete* in 2002.

In 1988, or 16 years after Wade's article appeared, *Science* published the standard claim but without any reference to Wade:

> The German government under Hitler developed and used [anabolic steroids], allegedly in an attempt to create an army of supermen.[39]

That same year, a newspaper in South Carolina reported that the Food and Drug Administration subscribed to the idea that the Nazis had used anabolic steroids to make German troops more aggressive.[40]

Reports about the mythical Nazi steroid continued throughout the 1990s and beyond, and not only in Taylor's works. In her pioneering book on the East German doping system, the former elite discus thrower, shot-putter and doping historian Brigitte Berendonk wrote in 1992:

> According to many survey articles, as early as the Second World War German Army [*Wehrmacht*] storm-troopers had been doped with testosterone for psychotropic purposes, only a few years after the first chemical identification, synthesis and determination of the structure of this compound.[41]

None of these sources were identified. Elsewhere in the book, Berendonk notes that 'androgenic military aggressiveness' had been recorded in writing by one research group as an area of interest, but without any reference to alleged Nazi interest in this topic.[42] A year later, the historian John Fair reported that Dr John Ziegler, who developed the anabolic steroid Methandrostenolone (Dianabol) for the CIBA pharmaceutical company (it was released in 1958), was provided by CIBA 'with books and records from Germany where similar experiments were carried out by the Nazis'.[43] In 2013, the author told us that his source had been the bodybuilder John Grimek, who:

> either saw these alleged books and records at Ziegler's office in Olney or that Ziegler told him about them. John liked to tell stories ... I actually worked in Ziegler's office and on his dining room table copying his correspondence on my old Remington typewriter, but I don't recall seeing (nor was I even looking for) materials of this kind.[44]

Once again, we see how unconfirmed or fanciful reports or mere impressions can work their way into an account in which the author's confidence in the reported information can seem more certain than it actually was. In 1999, Barry Houlihan wrote:

> The first medical use of the drug was in the 1930s when it was used to help the recovery of starvation victims. It was also used in the same decade for the non-medical purpose of increasing the aggressiveness and strength of German soldiers.[45]

Houlihan noted that 'much of this section uses Wadler G.I & Hainline, B. "Drugs and the Athlete" ... '.[46] As outlined above, Wadler and Hainline based their claim on Haupt and Roverc who, in turn, used Wade.[47] In 2001, Steven Ungerleider, an American sports psychologist, who was assisted by Brigitte Berendonk in the production of *Faust's Gold: Inside the East German Doping Machine*, wrote:

> During World War II, Hitler issued vast quantities of steroids to the SS and the Wehrmacht so that his troops would better resist combat fatigue and be more ruthless in following any order.

> As early as 1941, Soviet Red Army observers had noted an unusually passionate fighting spirit among German soldiers, who often seemed eager to die for the glory of the Third Reich.[48]

The author referred neither to sources nor to Berendonk's opinion on this matter.

Regarding the use of drugs for performance-enhancement in high-performance sport, we found a range of German publications from the 1920s and 1930s suggesting that drugs were used for performance-enhancement in sports.[49] As previously noted, there was even a case discussed at the congress of the Association of German Sports Physicians in 1927, where a doctor was accused of having administered injections to several high-performance athletes. In fact, the number of scientific publications dealing with the effects of pharmacological substances in the context of work and war, as well as the fact that scientifically based sports medicine developed earlier and more intensively in Germany than in any other country during this time, surely favoured athletes and doctors' experimentation with drugs in German sports.[50] However, regarding the Nazi Olympics of 1936, we don't have any empirical evidence that the Nazi regime systematically provided drugs to German athletes as the claim reported by Dimeo suggests. Furthermore, we don't have hard empirical evidence for testosterone use in sports during the interwar or Nazi periods. At first, testosterone was used to treat problems like fatigue, melancholia and impotence in older men, to deal with impotence in younger men, to treat testicular deficiency, to restore libido in women and to reverse homosexuality.[51] In fact, the Danish doctor Boje in 1939 appears to be the first to suggest that sex hormones might enhance physical performance.[52] Even in the first book on testosterone published in 1945, the author Paul de Kruif – a medical student during the 1920s and later a science reporter – presented its potential use in sports in only a few sentences and only as a future possibility.[53] The so-called 'Brustmann affair', in which the famous doctor Martin Brustmann administered testosterone to a German rowing team at the national Championships in 1952, appears to be the first well-documented case of testosterone use in sports in Germany.[54] The Brustmann affair is even earlier than the often-cited story about the US Olympic weightlifting coach Bob Hoffman and the team physician John Ziegler, who observed testosterone use by Soviet athletes at the 1952 Helsinki Olympic Games and the 1954 World Weightlifting Championships. Brustmann might have been inspired by a quite similar case two years earlier in which the Danish team physician Mathiesens had prescribed daily doses of the testicular extract Androstin to Danish rowers and which may constitute the first reliably documented case of the use of the male hormone in high-performance sport.[55]

Conclusion

Historical research on doping has to start with the ideas and concepts of those who were involved. Questions about how doping was defined, whether it was prohibited and whether it was prosecuted and sanctioned are crucial in this context. Briefly summarised, doping was morally offensive in amateur sports, but was rarely explicitly prohibited by formalised rules or prosecuted or sanctioned. Furthermore, it became increasingly unclear, due to rapid pharmacological developments, which other substances and methods apart from stimulants constituted doping. In fact, the question of whether the use of anabolic steroids constitutes doping was discussed openly until the 1970s.

We see no substantial evidence for the claim that German soldiers were given testosterone for performance-enhancement. The same applies to its use in sports during the Nazi period. There are only rumours or the uncritical repetition of previous and unsubstantiated claims.

Hoberman, Beamish and Ritchie have critically discussed the Nazi-steroid myth in some detail. They draw special attention to the role of rumours and stereotypes in this context. The myth of the Nazi steroid belongs to a larger category of rumours about the Nazis' willingness to use science in exotic ways for military purposes. Take, for example, the following *New York Times* report from 1944:

> It is said that the Nazis enable some of their fighter pilots to fly higher by removing part of the thyroid gland.[56]

Here, too, it is clear that the report is actually a rumour. It is also assumed that Nazi authorities are willing to mutilate their pilots to make them more effective, an idea that would have been compatible with contemporary reports of Nazi atrocities across Europe. In *The Hormone Quest* (1965), Albert Q. Maisel notes that research on the hormones of the adrenal cortex was considered high-priority research during the 1930s: 'But then World War II began, and all of these research teams were side-tracked into the search for the mythical steroid supposedly helping Nazi pilots to fly higher than our own'.[57]

This story was revived in 1993 in *Runner's World* magazine:

> Cortisone was discovered in the 1940s by scientists and physicians searching for a 'superhuman substance' reportedly in the hands of the Germans during World War II.[58]

Each of these reports confers on Nazi scientific activity a grotesque or magical quality: mutilation, a 'mythical steroid', a 'superhuman substance'.

Though it is true that Nazi soldiers used the amphetamine Pervitin during the war, the American and Japanese armies also consumed similar amphetamine drugs along with their German counterparts.[59] The fact that only Nazi soldiers have been associated with amphetamine and steroid use demonstrates the power of the Nazi stereotype. The Nazi steroid myth fits the image of the combat-ready German soldier and of Nazism as a masculine and aggressive ideology. Such stereotypical claims take oversimplified short cuts through a complex history. They seem convincing at first because stereotypical claims answer questions more quickly and clearly than differentiated views are ever able to do. Especially when claims seem to fit all too easily, critical historians should take a step back and focus attention on basic questions about what constitutes good historiography. Claims have to be substantiated by historical sources. Accordingly, our claim about the mythical nature of the Nazi steroid will be falsified only when and if historical documents appear which reliably show the contrary.

The persistence of the myth of the Nazi steroid, despite lacking empirical evidence, has to do with the over-credulous attitudes of otherwise competent and reliable commentators who seem to have applied less vigilance to this topic than they would apply to less sensational ones. It is worth noting that the myth of the Nazi steroid seems to have had only a minor career as a fringe doctrine on the Internet. It has rather persisted as a story that originated in a high-quality scientific publication and has been subsequently transmitted, or reported on, by respectable professionals such as physicians, academics and journalists.

In the last analysis, the myth of the Nazi steroid confirms the power of the Nazi myth itself, long after the eradication of the Third Reich. The sheer sadism of a criminal regime whose military power and racist fanaticism threatened to remake the world in its image continues to fascinate or obsess enormous numbers of people. A tiny minority of neo-Nazis continues to see Nazism as a doctrine of salvation for the white 'race' in general and for white males, in particular – hence the swastikas one sees on the jackets of motorcycle hoodlums around the world. Male domination in the Nazi style has set a standard no other masculine style has been able (or willing) to match. For masculine megalomania on this scale, only the male hormone will do.

Notes on Contributors

Marcel Reinold is a Ph.D. student and lecturer at the Institute for Sport and Exercise Sciences at the University of Münster (Germany). His research focuses on the history and sociology of doping and anti-doping policy.

John Hoberman is a professor at the Department of Germanic Studies at the University of Texas (Austin, USA). His research focuses on the history, sociology and politics of performance-enhancing substances in modern societies.

Notes

1. Paul Dimeo has refused to hammer the last nail into the coffin of the Nazi steroid myth: 'A number of writers have argued that steroids were manufactured and refined for physical performance purposes by the Nazi party during the Second World War. Houlihan offers the claim that steroids "were used [in the 1940s] for the non-medical purpose of increasing the aggressiveness and strength of German soldiers" (1999: 45). Unfortunately, he fails to cite any supporting evidence. John Hoberman discusses in some detail the myth of Nazi steroid science (1992) but it remains impossible to judge with any real certainty whether this myth has any basis in fact. There is no evidence available to support the claim. Regardless of the actuality, the myth does serve to support the broader association of steroids with exploitative, totalitarian regimes such as the Nazis, the German Democratic Republic and the Union of Soviet Socialist Republics'; see Dimeo, *A History of Drug Use*, 71–2.
2. Hoberman, *Mortal Engines*, 213–4.
3. See Hoberman, *Mortal Engines*, 216.
4. Dimeo, *A History of Drug Use*, 5.
5. See Reinold and Meier, "Difficult Adaptions to Innovations," 75.
6. See Worringen, "Doping im Sport"; Worringen, "Entgegnung"; Lade, "Anwendung ultravioletter Strahlen im Training"; and Hering, "Ultraviolette Strahlen für Sportzwecke."
7. Prokop, "Zur Geschichte des Dopings und seiner Bekämpfung," 130.
8. See Wilsdorf and Graf, "Historische Aspekte zur Entwicklung"; Gleaves, "Enhancing the Odds."
9. Deutsche Sportbehörde für Leichtathletik, *Wettkampfbestimmungen*, §32, point 7; Deutscher Reichsverband für Amateur-Boxen, *Wettkampfbestimmungen*, §30, point 11.
10. IAAF quoted in Vetteniemi, "Runners, Rumors, and Reams of Representations," 406. For early anti-doping movement in human sports, see also Gleaves, "Doped Professional and Clean Amateurs."
11. Ruhemann, "Verschiedenes," 36.
12. See Eckart, *Geschichte der Medizin*, 199–207.
13. Ibid., 268–83.
14. See Thoms, "Ernährung ist so wichtig wie Munition"; Neumann, "Ernährungsphysiologische Humanexperimente in der deutschen Militärmedizin."
15. See Ibid., 151–4.
16. See Stoff, *Wirkstoffe.*
17. Ibid., 30.
18. Ibid., 76.
19. See Thoms, "Ernährung ist so wichtig wie Munition," 216.
20. See Neumann, "Ernährungsphysiologische Humanexperimente in der deutschen Militärmedizin," 160–8.
21. See Roth, "Leistungsmedizin," 167–8.
22. Conti, quoted in Ibid., 171.
23. Drug regulations in Germany during that period did not aim at the prohibition of any type of drug but at the possession of drugs without a proper prescription. The first regulation against the trafficking with opiates and cocaine actually goes back to World War I. The German Opium Law of 1920 was a consequence of the Treaty of Versailles, which obliged Germany to ratify the International Opium Convention of 1912. Regulations changed during the 1920s. Finally, the Opium Law of 1929 incorporated previous regulations and created the possibility to include

new substances. Pervitin was included in the sixth amendment in 1941 due to its addictive nature. See Cousto, "Verbotene Früchte oder die Verordnungsflut," 204–6.

24. See Hoberman, *Mortal Engines*, 215.
25. Wade, "Anabolic Steroids," 1400.
26. Personal communication, April 8, 2013.
27. *The Male Hormone* was the title of a book published by the popular science writer Paul de Kruif in 1945. This well-researched manifesto on behalf of testosterone therapy for the aging male was widely reviewed, but the 55-year-old de Kruif did not achieve his goal of obtaining hormonal relief for his male cohort.
28. Baker, "Stop Blaming the Nazis."
29. Beamish and Ritchie, "Totalitarian Regimes and Cold War Sport," 25.
30. Haupt and Rovere, "Anabolic Steroids," 469.
31. Wadler and Hainline, *Drugs and the Athlete*, 56.
32. Perlmutter and Lowenthal, "Use of Anabolic Steroids," 208
33. Todd, "Anabolic Steroids," 93. Todd's footnote describing his sources is as follows:

    25. William Taylor, "The Case Against the Administration of HGH to Normal Children," presented at a symposium on *Ethical Issues in the Treatment of Children and Athletes with Human Growth Hormone*, University of Texas at Austin, April 26, 1986. Taylor's information on Hitler came from: "Hitler's Final Days," *American Medical News*, October 11, 1985, 1, 58–69. His source for the information on the storm troopers was Fred Silverman, "Guaranteed Aggression: The Secret Use of Testosterone by Nazi Troops," *Journal* of *the American Medical Association*, May 1984, 129–31.
34. A person named Fred Silverman was remembered in a paid notice in the November 8, 2001, issue of the *New York Times*:

    SILVERMAN – Frederick, M.D. Drs Barbara Edelstein and Kenneth Goldman mourn the passing of Dr. Fred Silverman. He was a doctor's doctor who served as a role model of honor, decorum and intellectual curiosity. He never considered night call an interruption of his evening activities, but the focus of his night. Dr. Silverman was a man of letters who could intelligently discourse and teach his companions on a wide variety of subjects from sports to ancient lore. Most importantly of all, Fred was a close friend whose company, with his wife Marilyn, we cherished. We will miss him.
35. Taylor, *Macho Medicine*, 8–9, 17. These comments are as follows: 'In the records of World War II are numerous accounts of hormonal manipulation and experimentation with human prisoners by Nazi scientists. After all, a group of German scientists pioneered the synthesis of testosterone and other hormones to follow. Several publications also suggest that testosterone and its analog, anabolic steroids, were given to Nazi troops to make them more aggressive in battle. But perhaps one of the first and certainly the most famous anabolic steroid user was Adolf Hitler From the records of Hitler's personal physician, it was reported that Hitler [8/9] was given injections of the "derivatives of testosterone" for a variety of presumed mental and physical ailments. In fact, besides the "derivatives of testosterone" (anabolic steroids), Hitler's physician reported that Hitler took methamphetamines and several other drugs now considered narcotics during his last few years of life. Who will ever know how much these psychoactive steroids and other narcotics affected Hitler's judgments and dehumanizing tactics? [8–9]

    Perhaps the German scientists, who were well ahead of their times partially due to their methods of human experimentation, would have a greater respect for the simple facts about testosterone therapy. But World War II came and dropped a curtain over German medical science, and the pioneering German hormone scientists faded from the scientific picture. German medical science was falling on evil days'. [17]

    Taylor offered the following comment later:

    'The ugliness of clinical experimentation with testosterone reared its head during World War II. In the records of this war are numerous accounts of hormonal manipulation and experimentation on human prisoners by Nazi [180/181] scientists. After all, a group of German research scientists pioneered the synthesis of testosterone and other hormones. They were awarded the Nobel Prize in medicine for it. Several anecdotal accounts have been published suggesting that testosterone and its analogs, anabolic steroids, were given to the Nazi Gestapo and Nazi troops to make them more muscular, sexually aggressive, and mean fighters in battle . . . '. Taylor, *Anabolic Steroids and the Athlete*.

36. Beamish, *Steroids*, 34–8.
37. Taylor, quoted in Ibid., 35.
38. Ibid.
39. Marshall, "The Drug of Champions," 183.
40. "Steroids Date Back at Least Half Century," *Spartanburg Herald-Journal*, November 11, 1988.
41. Berendonk, *Doping*, 241.
42. Ibid., 125.
43. Fair, "Isometrics or Steroids," 4.
44. Personal communication, April 2, 2013.
45. Houlihan, *Dying to Win*, 45.
46. Ibid.
47. Haupt and Rovere, "Anabolic Steroids"; Wade, "Anabolic Steroids."
48. Ungerleider, *Faust's Gold,* 45.
49. See Hoberman, *Mortal Engines*.
50. See Hoberman, "The Early Development of Sports."
51. See Hoberman, *Testosterone Dreams*, 114.
52. Yesalis and Bahrke, "Anabolic Steroid and Stimulant Use," 436.
53. de Kruif, *The Male Hormone*, 223.
54. See Reinold and Meier, "Difficult Adaptations to Innovations."
55. See "The Danish Oarsmen Who Took Part at the European Championships in Milan Were They Drugged?" *Bulletin du Comité International Olympique*, 28 (1951): 25–6.
56. "High Altitudes Via Chemicals: Gun-Shy Dogs and Neuroses," *New York Times*, April 16, 1944.
57. Maisel, *The Hormone Quest*, 95.
58. "Cortisone in Question," *Runner's World*, May 1993, 20.
59. Rasmussen, "Medical Science and the Military."

References

Baker, M. "Stop Blaming the Nazis for Steroids and Start Thanking the Jews." March 5, 2012. Accessed August 23, 2013. http://thinksteroids.com/articles/jews-nazis-steroids/

Beamish, R. *Steroids: A New Look at Performance-Enhancing Drugs*. Santa Barbara, CA: Praeger, 2011.

Beamish, R., and I. Ritchie. "Totalitarian Regimes and Cold War Sport: Steroid 'Übermenschen' and 'Ball-Bearing Females'." In *East Plays West: Sport and the Cold War*, edited by S. Wagg, and D. Andrews, 11–26. London: Routledge, 2007.

Berendonk, B. *Doping: Von der Forschung zum Betrug*. Reinbek: Rowohlt, 1992.

Cousto, H. "Verbotene Früchte oder die Verordnungsflut." In *Nazis on Speed: Drogen im Dritten Reich. Vol. 1.*, edited by W. Pieper, 204–208. Löhrbach: Edition Rauschkunde, 2002.

de Kruif, Paul. *The Male Hormone*. New York: Harcourt, Brace and Company, 1945.

Deutsche Sportbehörde für Leichtathletik. *Wettkampfbestimmungen*. München: Selbstverlag der D. S.B., 1927.

Deutscher Reichsverband für Amateur-Boxen. *Wettkampfbestimmungen*. München: Selbstverlag des D.R.f.A.B., 1929.

Dimeo, P. *A History of Drug Use in Sport: Beyond Good and Evil*. London: Routlegde, 2007.

Eckart, W. U. *Geschichte der Medizin. Fakten, Konzepte, Haltungen*. Berlin: Springer, 2009.

Fair, J. "Isometrics or Steroids? Exploring New Frontiers of Strength in the Early 1960s." *Journal of Sport History* 20, no. 1 (1993): 1–24.

Gleaves, J. "Doped Professional and Clean Amateurs: Amateurism's Influence on the Modern Philosophy of Anti-Doping." *Journal of Sport History* 38, no. 2 (2011): 237–254.

Gleaves, J. "Enhancing the Odds: Horse Racing, Gambling and the First Anti-Doping Movement in Sport, 1889–1911." *Sport in History* 32, no. 1 (2011): 26–52.

Haupt, H. A., and G. D. Rovere. "Anabolic Steroids: A Review of the Literature." *American Journal for Sports Medicine* 12, no. 6 (1984): 469–484.

Hering, W. "Ultraviolette Strahlen für Sportzwecke." *Die Leibesübungen* 13 (1926): 331.

Hoberman, J. "The Early Development of Sports Medicine in Germany." In *Sport and Exercise Science: Essays in the History of Sports Medicine*, edited by J. W. Berryman, and R. J. Park, 233–282. Urbana: University of Illinois, 1992.

Hoberman, J. *Mortal Engines: The Science of Performance and the Dehumanization of Sport*. New York: The Free Press, 1992.

Hoberman, J. *Testosterone Dreams: Rejuvenation, Aphrodisia, Doping*. Berkeley: University of California Press, 2005.

Houlihan, B. *Dying to Win*. Strasbourg: Council of Europe Press, 1999.

Lade, F. "Anwendung ultravioletter Strahlen im Training." *Die Leibesübungen* 2 (1926): 44.

Maisel, A. Q. *The Hormone Quest*. New York: Random House, 1965.

Marshall, E. "The Drug of Champions." *Science* 242, no. 4876 (1988): 183–184.

Neumann, A. "Ernährungsphysiologische Humanexperimente in der deutschen Militärmedizin 1939-1945." In *Medizin im Zweiten Weltkrieg. Militärmedizinische Praxis und medizinische Wissenschaft im 'Totalen Krieg'*, edited by W. U. Eckart, and A. Neumann, 151–170. Paderborn: Schöningh, 2006.

Perlmutter, G., and D. I. Lowenthal. "Use of Anabolic Steroids by Athletes." *American Family Physician* 32 (1985): 208–210.

Prokop, L. "Zur Geschichte des Dopings und seiner Bekämpfung." *Sportarzt und Sportmedizin* 21, no. 6 (1970): 125–132.

Rasmussen, N. "Medical Science and the Military: The Allies' Use of Amphetamine During World War II." *Journal of the Interdisciplinary History* 42, no. 2 (2011): 205–233.

Reinold, M., and H. E. Meier. "Difficult Adaptations to Innovations in Performance Enhancement: 'Dr. Brustmanns Power Pills' and Anti-Doping in German Post-War Sport." *Sport in History* 32, no. 1 (2012): 74–104.

Roth, K. -H. "Leistungsmedizin: Das Beispiel Pervitin." In *Ärzte im Nationalsozialismus*, edited by F. Kudlien, 167–174. Köln: Kiepenhauer & Witsch, 1985.

Ruhemann, W. "Verschiedenes." In *Muskelarbeit und Blutkreislauf. Verhandlungsbericht über die 4. Sportärztetagung in Berlin vom 22.–24. Oktober 1927*, edited by A. Mallwitz, and H. Rautmann, 34–37. Jena: Gustav Fischer, 1928.

Stoff, H. *Wirkstoffe. Eine Wissenschaftsgeschichte der Hormone, Vitamine und Enzyme 1920–1970*. Stuttgart: Franz Steiner Verlag, 2012.

Taylor, W. N. *Anabolic Steroids and the Athlete*. Jefferson, NC: McFarland Publishers, 2002.

Taylor, W. N. *Macho Medicine: A History of the Anabolic Steroid Epidemic*. Jefferson, NC: McFarland Publishers, 1991.

Thoms, U. "'Ernährung ist so wichtig wie Munition'. Die Verpflegung der deutschen Wehrmacht 1933–1945." In *Medizin im Zweiten Weltkrieg. Militärmedizinische Praxis und medizinische Wissenschaft im 'Totalen Krieg*, edited by W. U. Eckart, and A. Neumann, 207–229. Paderborn: Schöningh, 2006.

Todd, T. "Anabolic Steroids: The Gremlins of Sports." *Journal of Sport History* 14 (1987): 87–107.

Ungerleider, S. *Faust's Gold: Inside the East German Doping Machine*. New York: Thomas Dunne Books and St. Martin's Press, 2001.

Vetteniemi, E. "Runners, Rumors, and Reams of Representations." *Journal of Sport History* 37 (2010): 401–415.

Wade, N. "Anabolic Steroids: Doctors Denounce Them, But Athletes Aren't Listening." *Science* 176, no. 6 (1972): 1400.

Wadler, G. I., and B. Hainline. *Drugs and the Athlete*. Philadelphia, PA: F.A.A. Davis Company, 1989.

Wilsdorf, G., and G. Graf. "Historische Aspekte zur Entwicklung der Dopingforschung beim Pferd an der Veterinärmedizinischen Bildungsanstalt in Berlin 1925–1945." *Berliner Münchner Tierärztliche Wochenschrift* 111 (1998): 222–227.

Worringen, K. A. "Doping im Sport." *Die Leibesübungen* 14/15 (1926): 354–355.

Worringen, K. A. "Entgegnung auf die Äußerungen von Geh. Can.-Rat Dr. Hugo Bach." *Die Leibesübungen* 19 (1926): 448.

Yesalis, C. E., and M. S. Bahrke. "Anabolic Steroid and Stimulant Use in North American Sport Between 1850 and 1980." *Sport in History* 25, no. 3 (2005): 351–434.

The Emergence of Moral Technopreneurialism in Sport: Techniques in Anti-Doping Regulation, 1966–1976

Kathryn Henne

Regulatory Institutions Network, The Australian National University, Australia

This article focuses on the early work of the International Olympic Committee (IOC) Medical Commission's anti-doping policies as a unique form of moral entrepreneurship. As the concept suggests, the Medical Commission's rule-making power relied, in part, on members' expertise and their status as elites. It also came to depend upon technopreneurialism, that is, entrepreneurial scientific innovation, particularly in relation to methods of detecting evidence of doping. Attending to these distinctions, this article argues that these early efforts reveal the emergence of 'moral technopreneurialism'. By this, I refer to how technological developments serve and, in turn, shape anti-doping goals. Through an analysis of primary IOC documents and archival materials housed in Lausanne, Switzerland, this article considers how the Medical Commission implemented testing to detect evidence of doping from the mid-1960s through the 1976 Olympic Games in Montreal. These Games mark the introduction of anabolic steroids testing, which is noteworthy because the events leading up to it illustrate how policy-makers pushed for urgent scientific development, now an accepted trope in the fight against doping. This article concludes with a reflection on how technopreneurialism has culturally impacted the institutionalisation of the moral crusade against doping in sport.

Introduction

Sport, Paul Dimeo explains, is 'a technological process' of 'taking of a physical body and making it into something new in pursuit of athletic achievement', and doping, he argues, is 'only one more technological enhancement' to consider.[1] History supports his claim, as athletes and scientists have worked together in formal and informal capacities for over a century.[2] In the 1960s, anti-doping regulation was in part a response to concerns around the proliferation of 'unnatural' competitors, or, in other words, those athletes perceived to rely too strongly on artificial enhancement.[3] Almost ironically, science (in the form of testing for doping agents) emerged as the regulatory response to these technological anxieties. Pharmaceutical knowledge thus came to play an important role in both the enhancement of athletic performance and the regulation of performance enhancement.

Anti-doping policy has since been described as a form of 'technology-driven governance' that relies on scientific progress.[4] This article discusses how technologies have influenced not only the development of the International Olympic Committee's

(IOC) anti-doping policies and informed the trajectory of this regulation but also the cultural meanings attributed to and underpinning their justification. In doing so, my aim is to expand upon scholarly suggestions that 'moral entrepreneurship' has played – and continues to play – an important role in the development of drug testing and anti-doping policy.[5] Moral entrepreneurs, explains Howard Becker, promote their own normative values by ascribing a social label to a behaviour or practice through the creation or enforcement of rules that reflect and reinforce their own ideological disposition.[6] In this context, the embrace of technological innovation significantly shaped the nature and messages of moral entrepreneurship in this field. Within anti-doping regulation, technological innovation surpasses the technical refinement of testing procedures; it encompasses a broader set of creative and intellectual developments referred to as 'technopreneurialism'.[7] This commitment to innovation has come to anchor the regime and its pursuit of athletes using doping agents and methods. In fact, as I argue here, the interplay between scientific advances and the moral underpinnings of the anti-doping agenda has yielded a distinct process of *moral technopreneurialism*, which marks a paradigmatic shift from moral entrepreneurship.

While there are significant historical and social science analyses that recognise how political and ideological agendas influenced the deployment of scientific testing and procedures in this field, the cultural influence on science sometimes goes overlooked or underinterrogated. In this context, technologies are not simply 'things' shaped by social processes; they are cultural 'things' that also shape social processes. Science and technology studies (STS) scholars provide an important reminder that scientific pursuits of objective, seemingly 'law-like', truths are 'historical artefacts of instrumental reason'.[8] The use of technocratic tools as a response to cultural problems – like doping – hinges on an underlying belief in these 'truths'.[9] The regulation of doping in sport demonstrates a convergence between the cultures *of* science and the cultural beliefs justifying their intervention. In particular, it reveals how mobilising science aids in rendering moral claims as truth-claims, which Donna Haraway has explained as a technique that helps us to believe that these 'tricks' are essential facts.[10]

As the growing body of historical research on doping in sport attests, anti-doping practices and beliefs have taken shape as part of – and response to – broader transformations in modern sport. Fuelled by intense Cold War politics, the rise of highly developed national sport systems, accompanied by the professionalisation of sport and athletic performance training, relied strongly on scientific advances.[11] In fact, even though the arms race of the Cold War era no longer persists, there remains an arms race logic built into anti-doping regulation. Regulatory development is so closely linked to technopreneurial innovation that is often characterised as a competition between those developing (illegal) performance-enhancing substances and methods and those developing instruments to detect them. The establishment of the World Anti-Doping Agency (WADA) in 1999 and its subsequent technocratic expansion evidence how regulation hinges upon science and technology. This acceptance and normalisation of technopreneurialism have profoundly shaped the nature of anti-doping rules (i.e. their reliance on testing and surveillance mechanisms) and the framing of doping as a problem (i.e. as a dangerous cycle of innovating performance-enhancing methods).

Although many historians and social scientists have documented how medical experts shaped these developments, the few who examine science as a cultural influence on anti-doping regulation tend to focus on the contemporary proliferation of surveillance strategies, negating the important history of anti-doping efforts that predated the establishment of WADA.[12] This article, which draws primarily from sources housed in the

IOC Archives in Lausanne, Switzerland, revisits how anti-doping regulation took on a *scientistic* disposition and how developments in drug testing evidence it as a cultural shift.[13] In particular, it examines how advances in testing came to anchor and eventually drive anti-doping policy, thus offering historical insight into events that paved the way for contemporary anti-doping practices implemented by WADA.

To do so, this article revisits the formulation of anti-doping rules by the IOC Medical Commission, paying close attention how its members, most of whom were scientists, act as moral entrepreneurs. Moral entrepreneurship, a concept that has been applied usefully in relation to other anti-drug campaigns, captures how particular groups' lobbying efforts can lead to the institutionalisation of their moral agenda.[14] In short, their 'moral crusades', to use Becker's terminology, aim to make a practice a moral issue. Applying moral entrepreneurship to the issue of doping may illuminate that particular groups have lobbied to make it a morally condemnable offence; however, it does not provide a clear means through which to interrogate the role of science in advancing anti-doping policy. Scientific developments are more than tools leveraged by moral entrepreneurs against doping in sport; they are themselves actors that influenced moral entrepreneurs in this field and the rules they developed. Focusing on the first 10 years of the Medical Commission's work reveals how their efforts shifted to a technocratic focus that yielded a unique practice of legislating norms around performance enhancement and substance use. Although retaining core elements of moral entrepreneurship, these developments just as importantly demonstrate how technopreneurialism progressed and shaped the direction of the IOC's anti-doping platform.

The IOC Medical Commission's embrace of moral technopreneurialism crystallises around the development and implementation of a screening test that could detect whether athletes had used anabolic steroids in 1973. This article elucidates how scientific innovation became a prominent actor, exploring how advances simultaneously revealed and influenced the moral justifications of anti-doping policy. To illustrate relationships between moral claims and scientific developments, this analysis concentrates on how pressures to develop the tests for the metabolites of anabolic steroids influenced the IOC Medical Commission's work, the events around their implementation and the immediate aftermath of their inclusion. The conclusion then reflects on the legacies of these developments and how STS aids in making sense of science's longstanding cultural influenced on anti-doping regulation. In summary, it highlights how technopreneurialism in this field has served moral entrepreneurial agendas, eventually overshadowing a key moral impetus for anti-doping regulation: to protect athletes' health.

Understanding the IOC Medical Commission as a Moral Technopreneur

When developing and implementing anti-doping regulation, the Medical Commission operated in ways distinct from traditional notions of moral entrepreneurship. 'Rule creators', a category of moral entrepreneur described by Becker, are often portrayed as 'crusaders' championing a cause that they cast as a social threat.[15] Their work is typically to persuade others in society into accepting their perspective about the morality or immorality of a practice. If their crusade is successful, these values become institutionalised through the creation of new rules. Archetypal rule creators are ardent and sanctimonious, although they often see their cause as being for the greater social good. They, in turn, are not so much concerned with the details of the rules, but about pushing a reformist agenda. In extreme cases, the end results can serve to justify any means necessary.

Dimeo has similarly characterised some IOC Medical Commission members and other influential scientists during the 1960s and 1970s as 'proselytisers as well as fanatics' who sought to protect the purity of sport, not simply the health of athletes.[16] This coincided with a broader effort by Olympic officials to lobby for the international acceptance of sport as a distinct sphere because of its purity.[17] This notion of purity, though often attributed to having roots in Olympic principles such as amateurism, morphed as anti-doping regulation took shape.[18] At the time of the Medical Commission's establishment, the IOC and the Olympic Charter 'directly opposed the most extreme manifestations of the forces of scientific rationality and the cult of victory that increasingly threatened to undermine and debase the Olympic project'.[19] In essence, this stance assumed that practices of doping embodied the values of 'pursuing winning at all costs', undermining the Olympic principles of camaraderie and moral development cultivated by amateur sport. Anti-doping regulation emerged as a tool to protect core Olympic values, but the competitive climate of Cold War sport, increasingly sophisticated scientific tools and the wider professionalisation of sport would come to undermine and change the purpose and principles of the Olympic movement.

By focusing on scientific testing, the IOC Medical Commission's proselytising took on decidedly secular and apolitical contours. While Medical Commission members' personal correspondence and other writings reveal deeper moral beliefs for condemning doping, their enduring acts of moral entrepreneurship take on a technocratic form.[20] In clinging to objective measures, the Medical Commission's recommendations seemingly disavow cultural factors; however, this erasure is an important aspect of science's cultural influence: those developing and deploying these tools have an 'unmarked' power 'to see and not be seen'.[21] By leveraging drug testing to preserve bodily (and presumably moral) purity, regulation has rendered the cultural tenets of amateurism as tangible truth-claims, not as a forthright ideological stance. In other words, the basis of testing suggests that bodies *can and should be* natural. However, recognising sport as a technological process reveals that drug testing actually only distinguishes some methods of performance enhancement as amoral. In a very basic sense, science influences how anti-doping regulation levies its moral claims, doing so in ways that are often discursive and not always rendered explicit.

Well before scholars characterised the Medical Commission as a group of moral entrepreneurs, critical commentators referred to their work as a 'crusade'. For instance, in describing the anti-doping 'crusade', sports doctor Lan Barnes explained that anti-doping policies were flawed, yet nonetheless growing. Dominated by European doctors, the anti-doping effort, he argued, used a variety of reasons to justify its cause, including that doping caused 'physiological damage, addiction, psychological deterioration, and progressive moral degradation'.[22] Pointing to the limitations of regulatory tactics, he stressed that 'the list of banned drugs and practices they recommend is only limited by the availability of tests for the substance'.[23] Barnes thus highlighted an underlying tension: relying on scientific testing only addressed elements of the doping problem. Rules were only as robust as the science that underpinned them, which perpetuated a cycle of necessary innovation in order to detect more doping products and agents. This limitation, now an embedded feature of anti-doping regulation, was the outgrowth of the Medical Commission's regulatory interventions, which had taken on a distinctly technocratic focus as early as 1967.

Depending primarily upon drug testing was not the evident course of action when the IOC began formal discussions of regulating drugs in sport. Although IOC members condemned doping in the Olympic Games as early as 1937, it did not emerge as a pressing concern until the 56th IOC Session in 1960.[24] In San Francisco, President Avery Brundage raised the issue, focusing on the use of amphetamines, or 'pep pills'.[25] During the meeting, the prospect of endorsing the scientific examination of doping arose but was not pursued. Instead, members were only encouraged to 'speak of this matter in their respective countries'.[26] Months later, however, the death of Danish cyclist Knud Jensen during the Rome Olympics emphasised the need for regulation. While it prompted the IOC Executive Board to call for sanctions, the IOC again failed to take action.[27] Having reportedly taken stimulants prior to the race, Jensen's death became symbolic by seemingly demonstrating that athletes needed to be saved from the dangers, both moral and physical, inherent to the 'winning at all costs' mentality promoted by professional sport.[28] Accompanying this aversion to professional sport and its technologies of performance enhancement was also a hesitation by the IOC Executive Board to embrace – and fund – scientific testing to enhance its regulatory response to doping.[29]

The IOC Medical Commission did not began its work on scientific testing and protocols until 1967 after its first Chairperson, Sir Arthur Porritt (who had served for six years, yet accomplished little in terms of policy), stepped down to accept his appointment as the Governor-General of New Zealand. Only two months after his departure, British champion Tom Simpson became another high-profile cyclist whose death was attributed to the use of stimulants during competition. Porritt's position on what constitutes doping and how to counteract it is notably different from contemporary rhetoric.[30] Defining doping, he argued, 'is, if not impossible, at best extremely difficult, and yet everyone who takes part in competitive sport or who administers it knows exactly what it means. The definition lies not in words but in integrity of character'.[31] Porritt also stressed that 'only a long-term education policy stressing the physical and moral aspects of the drug problem' would prevent and deter athletes from using ergogenic aids.[32] Connecting the physical and the moral aspects of sport reflected foundational Olympic principles. As Rob Beamish and Ian Ritchie write, 'The overly competitive zeal represented by the use of performance-enhancing substances fell outside the Movement's moral code. This was the educational message Porritt wanted conveyed to the athletes of the Games'.[33]

Porritt's tenure as the Medical Commission's Chairman was marked by inaction, though. Evidence suggests that he was not simply hesitant to act, but perhaps disinterested as he sometimes failed to attend meetings and submit reports.[34] The Medical Commission did not deliver its first report until 1966, over five years after its establishment. Reflecting Porritt's normative focus, it suggested the following recommendations as the basis of anti-doping efforts:

(1) National Olympic Committees (NOCs) should begin work on general education;
(2) the inclusion of entry forms signed by competitors with a statement that he or she did not dope (which would pave the way for testing and examinations);
(3) international federations should prohibit the behaviour in their own rules;
(4) the IOC should formally condemn doping and sanction either NOCs or individual athletes if found guilty of an offence during the Olympic Games and
(5) it should ensure that testing can take place when deemed necessary.

While this early articulation of the Medical Commission's position embraced fundamental tenets of moral entrepreneurship by promoting the broader condemnation of doping in sport, its initial lack of follow-through made it far from a fervent crusader. Beyond Porritt's own reluctance, the IOC did not participate in the first conference on the subject of doping, which was held by Council of Europe (CoE) in 1963.

Taking action without the IOC, the CoE Commission worked out a distinctly different notion of doping. It defined doping as:

> the administration to or the use by, a competing athlete of any substance foreign to the body or any physiological substance taken in abnormal quantity or by an abnormal route of entry into the body, with the sole intention of increasing in an artificial and unfair manner his performance in competition.[35]

The CoE Commission's definition married moral and physiological concerns. It made the direct connection that the presence of a 'foreign' (and presumably unnatural) substance in an athlete's body marked an ethical transgression. Interestingly, the definition did not explicitly address physical well-being, even though health risks served as a direct impetus for developing anti-doping policy. Nonetheless, this definition labelled doping an act of deviance, providing the grounds to justify drug testing as a way to obtain evidence of an athlete's transgression. This definitional act did more than condemn doping; it set the stage for rules and sanctions based on the findings of testing. It enabled technology to serve as the mechanism through which to inscribe a cultural belief in the virtue of bodily purity, which values of amateurism already supported. The ability to detect a substance presented an otherwise ideological claim more tangible by providing an empirical mechanism to 'prove' the presence of an impure substance.

The IOC Medical Commission later embraced the tenets of the CoE Commission's definition under the Chairmanship of Porritt's replacement, Prince Alexandre de Mérode of Belgium. In pursuing this narrow, albeit still vague, definition of doping, the Medical Commission's work took on an explicitly technocratic focus under de Mérode, but it did not depart from ideological foundations. The adoption of a technocratic focus is not surprising given that seven of the other members appointed to the Commission were specialists in either medicine or pharmacology. In fact, other than de Mérode, only Arpad Csanadi of Hungary lacked training in these fields. The other members were Dr Arnold Beckett of Great Britain; Dr Albert Dirix, Vice President of the Belgian Olympic Committee; Dr Roger Genin of France who was also on the Organising Committee of the 1968 Olympic Games in Grenoble; Eduardo Hay, the Medical Director of the 1968 Olympic Games in Mexico; Professor Giuseppe La Cava, the President of the International Federation of Sports Medicine; Professor Ludwig Prokop of Austria; and Pieter Van Dijk, President of the Medical Commission of the International Cycling Union.[36] Dirix and Prokop had been part of a group that had met and arranged small-scale testing at the 1964 Tokyo Games, while Beckett had aided in the development of procedures and rules for the 1966 football World Cup.[37]

Apart from their collective expertise, many of these appointees had also expressed strong anti-doping sentiments, some of which focused on the issue of athletes' health and others on ethical concerns. For instance, La Cava had written that amphetamines' performance-enhancing effects were 'illegitimate' in terms of ethics and dangerous in terms of health.[38] Prokop too had cast doping as an immoral act while attending the CoE Commission conference. Having encountered amphetamine use among cyclists he treated, he had denounced the sport's resistance to anti-doping efforts and later argued that sports doctors often enabled drug use.[39] Attributing Jensen's death to doping, Dirix had appealed, 'We doctors wish to prevent such tragedies'. Characterising doping as a widespread 'evil', he explained that 'nothing could be more criminal than to destroy the health or life of a young athlete'.[40]

Although many members justified their work in moral terms, a series of technocratic priorities that 'placed a particular emphasis on medical controls concerning both doping and the establishment of sex' emerged from the Medical Commission's first meeting in September 1967.[41] The five areas of the concern were:

(1) the need for entry forms requiring athletes and NOCs to consent to medical examinations 'thought necessary in the interests of both his health and future';
(2) the development of a list of banned substances as well as sample collection and laboratory testing procedures;
(3) the random selection of athletes for anti-doping testing and mandatory sex testing of the three winning female competitors;
(4) the obligation of international federations to disseminate information in order to ease implementation and
(5) the provision of medical assistance to any country who does not have adequate staff at either the 1968 Grenoble or Mexico City Games.[42]

Focussing on the implementation of medical protocols required the involvement of Commission members, which the Commission's earlier recommendations under Porritt's chairmanship did not endorse. Of these revised goals, the second and aspects of the third became the central focus of the Medical Commission's work, especially in its early years. Thus, as early as 1967, the direction of the Medical Commission's work would follow a decidedly scientific path.

As a collective, the Medical Commission was not only a 'rule creator' but also a 'rule enforcer', which are two distinct categories of moral entrepreneurs under Becker's original explanation. In fact, Becker described rule enforcers as part of the development of organisations and rules that resulted from successful moral crusades led by reformers.[43] Because of its members' medical expertise, the Medical Commission wore both hats, often simultaneously. As 'rule creators', members gave credence to anti-doping guidelines because their collective social status and scientific training lent credibility to regulatory claims and tools. They were also sometimes 'rule enforcers' who carried out the tests and made decisions on punishment, although this changed later as anti-doping regulation expanded. The rules and membership of the Medical Commission would fluctuate in the years that followed; however, de Mérode and Beckett would directly influence anti-doping policy for more than three decades. While Beckett's suggestions for testing procedures and methods impacted the actual protocols carried out, the Prince was the more active lobbyist – at least early on. In fact, de Mérode – who has been criticised as an ineffective Chairman by some[44] – made up for his lack of formal medical training by advocating on behalf of the Medical Commission. His contributions, which I further explain in the next section, ensured that it became a recognised voice within the Olympic Movement.

Early Drug Testing under the IOC Medical Commission

Focusing on the technical aspects of outlining the methods of testing and analysis, the Medical Commission agreed to use thin-layer and gas chromatography.[45] Members also decided upon five classifications of banned substances, which were notably few compared to the thousands of individual substances currently banned by WADA. They were sympathomimetic amines; stimulants of the central nervous system (strychnine) and analeptics; narcotics and analgesics; anti-depressants, imipramine and similar substances; and major tranquilisers.[46] Recognising their limitations, the members of the Medical Commission included a clause acknowledging, 'We have concentrated on products which are detrimental when used by healthy athletes in competition, but which on the other hand are used for therapeutic reasons'.[47] The initial list of banned substances therefore reflected athletes' health and well-being as primary concerns.

One notable exception to the list of banned substances was anabolic steroids. Amphetamines had been the primary focus of the Medical Commission's work prior to de Mérode's Chairmanship, even though, as Beckett later stated, members were aware of the steroids use as early as 1960.[48] In order to detect them and other substances, the development and oversight of testing protocols took precedence; however, the process of implementing protocols, or even establishing the Medical Commission's credibility, was not smooth or uncontested. As Steven Epstein acknowledges, credibility is itself a process, one that is 'both a stake and a weapon in the skirmishes between all those who are in competition' as well as a 'mechanism for forging durable relationships within which knowledge can reliably be exchanged'.[49] An early battle regarding the role of the Medical Commission offers an illustration of this point: the Prince faced direct challenges from President Brundage who, concerned with the IOC's finances (or lack thereof), did not feel that the IOC should shoulder the responsibility of implementing drug testing procedures. Specifically, in a circular to international sport federations, NOCs and IOC members dated August 27, 1968, Brundage (without consulting de Mérode) announced that the Commission's role was merely advisory in nature.

At the time of the distribution of Brundage's letter, the Medical Commission had already developed testing protocols that required its members' direct involvement. In fact, the Medical Commission had delineated its duties, which were to:

> carry out the taking of the urine samples on a random basis and the laboratory analysis. In addition, in the case of doubt, they must decide whether a misuse has been made of the dope substances and, each time, a positive result is obtained, advise the authorized disciplinary department accordingly in a strictly confidential manner. The Medical Commission should meet every two days [during the Games]. Should positive results be obtained during the dope test or other questions, such as those pertaining to the sex tests for example, arise, it should meet as soon as possible.[50]

Responsibilities and testing procedures had been outlined, which prompted the Prince to respond directly to Brundage, copying all parties who received the original memorandum. Calling Brundage's letter 'a serious blow to the work we are trying to achieve', he wrote that the role of the Commission had been defined and 'cannot be changed unilaterally without first consulting the qualified authorities who decreed them', adding that 'these extremely delicate matters concern the moral responsibility of the IOC and go far beyond technical questions, if we still wish to remain loyal to the fundamental principles of the Olympic Spirit'.[51]

In terms of the genealogy of moral technopreneurialism in this space, de Mérode's argument was important, because it highlighted that technical procedures should not overshadow or erase the normative reasons for anti-doping regulation. In fact, de Mérode's argument contended that they could be complimentary. Not only did this mark an attempt to assuage IOC members' anxieties around technology, it actually refigured Olympic values in a way that rendered them compatible with scientific pursuits. Although disagreeing with and defying Brundage, he did so by appealing to Olympic agendas. This development emerged as part of a broader shift within the Olympic Movement, which moved away from the formal doctrine of amateurism towards principles that reconciled ongoing changes in sport sparked by professionalism and increasingly competitive sporting systems.[52] De Mérode's words nonetheless struck a balance by articulating the place of the Medical Commission within the values upon which the Olympic Movement hinged. Brundage would clarify his position, writing that he had 'no intention whatsoever on my part to undermine the Medical Commission'. He specified, 'If there is any testing done in Mexico, it will be done under the supervision of this Commission and according to its regulations and procedures. However, it must be done at the written request of the International Federations concerned'.[53]

Beyond these initial conflicts, difficulties arose during the 1968 Olympic Games in Grenoble. French laboratories, for instance, could not manage all of the analyses, having only been reminded five days before the beginning of the competition that they were to carry out tests, 'and of course, in this minimal time, they were not able to establish a sufficiently equipped laboratory to deal with the technical requirements of these tests'.[54] Further, then, 'counter-checking' the samples was not possible on site: if an athlete suspected of doping had requested his or her second sample be tested (as it was not compulsory), Beckett would have had to conduct the analysis at his laboratory in London.[55] With no positive tests, this was not an issue; however, the (lack of) findings cast doubt on the effectiveness of testing. Reporting on drug tests conducted at the Games, Dr Jacques Thiébault indicated, 'This is the first time such action has been taken at the Olympic Games, which accounts for certain imperfections on the practical side of these controls, which should, however, be easily eliminated in the future'.[56] Although there were improvements in Mexico City, the Medical Commission was still aware it needed to improve protocols and ensure that more athletes were tested. Capacity building became important: there was only one three-room medical facility at the Mexico City Games (with a room each dedicated to reception, administration and testing), and the report filed on both Grenoble and Mexico City Games suggested the need for more on-site help from trained medical staff.[57]

In an attempt to standardise procedures, the Commission published its first pamphlet in 1972, which contained clearer rules, procedures and sanctions, as well as a direct statement on the Medical Commission's purpose. This publication articulated a message that has come to anchor anti-doping rhetoric: science would protect the showcasing of athletes' natural abilities, a value previously guarded by the Olympic Charter and its amateurism requirements (which were struck from the Charter's text in 1974). Competitors also received 'green cards', which, like the US naturalisation documents of the same nickname, essentially allowed them to 'legally' enter the Olympic Games. Testing and documentation certified them as eligible competitors, providing technocratic mechanisms to enforce the Olympic Charter's explicit condemnation of 'the use of drugs or artificial stimulants of any kind'.

Amidst the growing awareness of athletes using drugs other than amphetamines and in sports beyond cycling, an endorsement of the Medical Commission's importance came from Brundage's successor, Lord Killanin, who described 'doping as one of the greatest problems of the Olympic Movement', stating that purpose of the Medical Commission was to 'strive as far as it can against the creation of the artificial man or woman'.[58] Other researchers have explained that this statement marked a shift in thinking about doping in which 'steroids presented the new problem of altering human physiology'.[59] Construed as not simply cheating, but as 'playing God', the stakes appeared much higher, and the need for swift and severe action seemed pressing, marking the beginning of an accepted arms race mentality.[60] Technological expectations, as part of the cultural conditions of scientific mobilisation via anti-doping regulation and competitive sporting regimes, directly informed the allegory and the regulatory response it called for: stronger anti-doping capacities enabled by technopreneurialism. This change reiterated the importance of both testing and sanctions, and it revealed a subscription to two kinds of competing technologies: one used unfairly to modify athletes' bodies – a kind of 'bad', unethical science – and one leveraged to regulate these forms of enhancement – a presumably 'good', counteractive science. A notion of purity rooted in bodily and moral integrity still justified anti-doping protocols, but the discourse had shifted, overshadowing the moral concerns around athletes' health. No longer was doping criminal to the athletes, as Dirix had once explained; rather, doping athletes emerged as unnatural and thus criminal.

Given the limitations of drug testing, the Medical Commission's certification process did not ensure that all competitors were, in fact, uncontaminated by 'foreign' substances. Rumour, speculation and anecdotal evidence supported fears that steroid use had become widespread in order for competitors to catch up with East German athletes suspected of systematically doping.[61] With the Soviet Union replicating the German Democratic Republic's centrally planned approach to elite athlete development and both Communist countries providing financial support, there was additional pressure for Western countries to better organise their athlete development programming – and for their athletes to use doping methods to remain competitive.[62] The Medical Commission, in turn, strongly condemned steroid use, but it could not test for the metabolites at the time of the Games held in 1968 and 1972.

Developing and Implementing a Test for Steroids Metabolites

With the rules themselves – not just their enforcement – dependent on science's ability to detect banned substances, the development of an effective test for steroids became a growing concern as there was evidence of widespread steroid use by the late 1960s and at the 1972 Olympics, including an unofficial poll finding that two-thirds of athletes from a variety of countries (USA, USSR, UK, Canada, Egypt, New Zealand and Morocco) and sports had used steroids during the lead-up to those Games.[63] Dimeo explains that prior to the introduction of a test, there was 'little ethical debate among athletes' regarding their use.[64] Further, and in part 'due to the sportive nationalism catalysed by the Cold War', argue Thomas Hunt, Paul Dimeo and Scott Jedilicka, 'neither side of the Iron Curtain wanted to cause a disadvantage to their athletes by pushing for an effective anti-doping regime'.[65] Smaller countries too had become swept up in the sports arms race. For example, New Zealand team doctor T.R. Anderson contended that the use of anabolic steroids was especially common in strength sports. Writing to IOC Director Monique Berlioux, he explained, 'Their [Steroids'] harmful effects are known, but not yet fully understood, and I would suggest that while champion performance depends on these drugs, participants in these events be excluded from future New Zealand teams'.[66] In other words, Anderson appealed for the banning of his own nation's strength athletes under the presumption that every one of them used anabolic steroids.

Writing on behalf of the Medical Commission, Beckett reflected that 'the banning of the use of anabolic steroids was considered to be necessary even in 1967', but there was no test to support the enforcement of such a prohibition.[67] When the UK Sports Council announced in late 1973 that a research team had 'progressed to a stage' at which it could test blood and urine samples to detect whether athletes had taken anabolic steroids, the Medical Commission welcomed the development.[68] To justify the prohibition of anabolic steroids, Beckett evoked health-related concerns:

> By 1974, sufficient progress [in terms of testing] had been made for the IOC Medical Commission to include anabolic steroids in the list of prohibited drugs at the Olympic Games. Anabolic steroids are compounds which represent chemical modifications of the male hormone testosterone in which the anabolic effect, i.e. the muscle building actions are enhanced ... The reason for banning them is not only because their use contravenes

> sporting ethics but because it constitutes a definite danger to females and also to the growth of young people; furthermore, the use of some anabolic steroids in large doses may cause liver damage, affect spermetogenisis [sic] and there are reports of their use constituting a cancer hazard.[69]

Beckett's statements about the effects of steroids, however, were not universally supported – at least not in the way that his language may seem to suggest. There were ongoing scientific studies about how to discern the physiological effects of anabolic steroids use, many of which resulted mixed findings, especially in relation to health consequences.[70] In fact, one of the scientists who worked on the UK Sports Council-funded project aimed at developing detection techniques, Professor Prutny, acknowledged there was a lack of evidence, positing that such risks were likely reversible after discontinuing use.[71]

There were also questionable tactics being used to deter the use of anabolic steroids, even by medical professionals aligned with the IOC. US medical doctor Daniel Hanley (who had become a member of the IOC Medical Commission) reportedly told athletes that steroids had a placebo effect. In an interview, US high jumper Chris Dunn publically criticised Hanley's method:

> How are athletes supposed to take the drug problem seriously when the alleged 'experts' like Dr Hanley tell all the Olympic weight men to their faces that steroids only help psychologically – when every weight man on the U.S. team took them? Steroids are wrong, but you can't curb an athlete from taking them by lying to his face.[72]

Not only did Dunn reject Hanley's claims, but his antipathetic words suggest he was insulted by Hanley's 'lying' about the widespread recognition of anabolic steroids' performance-enhancing benefits.

Regardless of these debates, when the UK Sports Council announced in 1973 that, after four years of research, a team led by Professor Brooks at St Thomas's Hospital Medical School in London indicated that it had developed a screening test that could 'detect whether sports competitors have been taking anabolic steroids, although to obtain conclusive evidence of the particular drug it might be necessary to use mass spectrometry techniques'.[73] Following the news, the Chairman of the British Sports Council, Roger Bannister, provided additional information after meeting with Beckett:

> Professor Beckett accepts that this test is a satisfactory screening-test but his Commission has always required back-up proof of identification of the precise chemical (in this case it could be one of some 15 variants on the anabolic theme) before they would ban an athlete. This is possible for some drugs by the rather expensive technique of mass spectrometry (equipment costing £50,000) and some research yet to come.[74]

He continued, writing that 'with international backing, these tests could most certainly be developed over the next year or so, well in time for Montreal'.[75] Even without compelling evidence of a threat to athletes' health, the IOC Medical Commission sought to implement the test. As other scholarly accounts have illustrated, Cold War rhetoric and anxieties around the growing number of seemingly unnatural athlete bodies, particularly those competing in women's events, coalesced to fortify its justifications.[76] This instance of technopreneurialism marked how foundational moral claims had begun to shift in relation to social changes and scientific developments.

Accompanying the test in 1974, the IOC amended its rules to ban not only competitors found to have doping agents in their system but also 'any athlete refusing to take a doping test'.[77] This rendered any athlete unwilling to comply or resistant towards compliance a transgressor. In 1975, the IOC supported a formal stance that 'doping is forbidden', stating that it was responsible for developing the banned substances list and that the Medical

Commission was to develop rules of application and implement them. Technological development had therefore actually contributed to changing the definitions and meanings of what it was to be an eligible Olympic athlete. For Beamish and Ritchie, these developments coincided with the 'watershed' of the Olympic Movement, which revealed that 'the constitutive practices of world class, high performance sport were finally, and resolutely, undermining [Pierre] de Coubertin's cardinal principles'.[78] High-performance sport had changed the Olympics, and the rules, which were backed and enabled by technological techniques, reflected these shifts.

The Medical Commission indeed endorsed the procedures for the 1976 Olympic Games after a trial of random testing at the 1975 Commonwealth Games yielded nine positive results for steroids out of 55 samples (two of which were randomly selected for a more detailed examination using gas–liquid chromatography–mass spectrometry, which confirmed them as positive).[79] In total, there were 2001 tests conducted at the Games held in Montreal, 268 targeting anabolic steroids.[80] There were, however, expressed reservations regarding the implementation of specific tests for anabolic steroids metabolites. James Worrall, a Canadian IOC Member, wrote directly to de Mérode, providing the following explanation for his resistance to such testing:

> Present evidence would appear to indicate that testing for steroids is quite inconclusive and the effect of the use of such drugs could be very easily circumvented by any athlete who has been taking them, by merely discontinuing the use of them for a reasonable period prior to competition. It is also indicated that the technical requirements for setting up a depot for steroid testing are going to be extremely expensive, both from an equipment and personnel requirement standpoint.[81]

This challenge was distinctly different from Brundage's claims in 1968. Instead of questioning the Medical Commission's authority or the place of testing, Worrall accepted both. Instead, his concern focused on doubts that testing was not yet accurate or sophisticated enough to justify the financial burden accrued through implementation. Thus, even in protest, Worrall's words revealed a tacit acceptance of the future capabilities of anti-doping technologies, not questioning whether innovation would eventually deliver an accurate test for steroids metabolites worth the associated financial costs.

Overall, testing at the 1976 Games in Montreal yielded findings for 11 disqualifications: 3 resulting from the use of various substances (competitors in weightlifting, shooting and yachting) and 8 stemming from the detection of anabolic steroids use (1 in athletics, 7 in weightlifting) and 3 resulting from the use of other substances (competitors in weightlifting, shooting and yachting).[82] There were, however, problems with regard to results management, some of which were grave administrative errors. One, in particular, led to the mishandling of the positive tests. In fact, the press reported the names of five athletes who tested positive prior to the accused being informed. As recounted by the then President of the International Weightlifting Federation (IWF), Gottfried Schödl:

> On the late evening of the 10th of August 1976 I was phoned by Mr. Oscar State [former IWF General Secretary] from London. He informed me that there are five weightlifters with positive results on anabolic steroids in the first analysis of doping. He gave me the names ... On the 12th of August 1976 I could read the names of those five weightlifters in a German paper. The same day I was informed with cable by Mr. Dirix [of the Medical Commission] about these doping cases but without names. This was the correct way. According to the rules there is only one person who has to be informed in cases of positive doping results: the President of the competent federation.[83]

At the time, State was not an IWF official, and Schödl expressed his disappointment in the Medical Commission members' 'indiscreetness', which caused 'damage not only to five weightlifters reputation before an official IOC decision but also to IWF's reputation'.[84]

Over the next two months, controversy ensued around the events that led to the disclosure of information and, as a result of the indiscretion, how to handle the athletes' cases. The respective national governing bodies of three of the accused weightlifters also filed complaints alleging that sample containers had been opened in transit as well (which was denied).[85] At the Medical Commission meeting held that October in Barcelona, members resolved the issue. Because the tests were positive, the athletes would be disqualified, despite the petitions regarding procedural irregularities. These developments reflected the recognition that the Medical Commission had decision-making, even quasi-juridical, authority embedded in its technocratic role. This was despite its members' violation of their own stated principles and commitments to confidentiality. Despite possible inconsistencies in managing the samples and challenges from governing bodies, the Medical Commission's decisions also still held. Irrespective of its shortcomings, the Medical Commission occupied a much more secure place within the Olympic Movement than it had 10 years prior, in large part because of de Mérode's early lobbying efforts and the influence of scientific testing.

Concluding Remarks on Moral Technopreneurialism After 1976

Following the 1976 Olympiad, the Medical Commission continued to expand its capacity. The Medical Commission no longer needed to lobby to secure its place within the moral crusade against doping. Instead, its work focused on technocratic improvements and research to enhance testing. The numbers of banned substances continued to increase as technological developments enabled testing for more compounds, as would budgets for testing facilities.[86] Commenting on these efforts, Dimeo, Hunt and Bowers suggest that 'an implied fear of change, modernity, and over-use of technological forms of enhancement' underpinned these developments, even though there was 'no evidence of widespread usage and no challenge to the ongoing obsession with winning'.[87] It would appear, then, that an emergent embrace of technopreneurialism had a clear, arguably agentive, role in setting the anti-doping agenda.

In the short term, improving on-site testing facilities and meeting these requirements increased costs and burdens to international federations and host cities, most urgently to Lake Placid and Moscow, the sites of the 1980 Olympic Games. Possibly undermined by financial demands, there was little information dispersed about testing following those Games. There were no positive tests reported in Lake Placid, even though it is speculated that 440 tests were conducted, 350 targeting anabolic steroids.[88] There were also no positive tests at the 1980 Summer Games in Moscow, even though 2488 tests were conducted, 800 targeting anabolic steroids.[89] Likely spinning these shortcomings in a positive light, de Mérode declared the 1980 Moscow Games to be the most 'pure' in Olympic history.[90] Despite this claim, he and the Medical Commission continued to outline additional needs, which included provisions to unify approaches, procedures and rules among international federations and to establish a network of accredited laboratories.[91] These proposals later became integral components of the current anti-doping regime under WADA. Underpinned by technopreneurial drives, these developments paved the way for a professionalised anti-doping bureaucracy. As the institutionalised embodiment of the moral crusade during the 1960s and 1970s, there are now a host of rule enforcers who have followed the Medical Commission and modified the techniques of anti-doping regulation.

As those subsequent shifts have been detailed by historians and social scientists elsewhere, my conclusion here focuses on how a scientistic logic became culturally reinscribed in a way that made moral entrepreneurship in this field distinctly different than

Becker's typology. In this context, it has yielded a cyclical process: as anti-doping regulation secured more technological techniques in response to growing pressures, rules and discourse shifted, requiring the nature of the Medical Commission's moral entrepreneurship to also adapt. Originally posited as a defender of athlete's health and sport's ethics, regulatory techniques have translated the notion of bodily purity (as an engrained value to protect) into the pursuit of a detectable impurity in the form of doping metabolites. This embedded belief has come to anchor the justification for regulation and the perpetual scientific development encouraged by the arms race mentality directed at doping athletes. Like the prevailing Cold War rivalries in international sport, this mentality relies upon the culture of technopreneurialism, which has become institutionalised.

The Medical Commission's development from 1966 to 1976 highlights how technocratic rules and technological techniques directly informed cultural shifts in sport. In this case, the ability to see athletes suspected of doping with the naked eye, but not the actual biological impurity (presumed to cause the visible abnormality), reinforced a dependency upon sample collection and testing that supported the Medical Commission's moral crusade. To counteract doping more effectively, testing innovations sought to detect more doping agents. In doing so, they substantiated the need for enhancing technological instruments by providing evidence to support suspicions of athletes' impure behaviours. Thus, rather being a testament of linear scientific progress pursing a scientific truth, anti-doping efforts emerge as a cycle, the beginning of which crystallised around the Medical Commission feeling compelled to innovate technologies of testing in order to catch athletes using steroids.

Today, an arms race mentality is embedded in the anti-doping regime, as evidenced by WADA's expanding use of testing and surveillance technologies. WADA has established the online Anti-Doping Administration & Management System; developed the Whereabouts programme in order to collect samples from athletes without providing advance notice; introduced the Biological Passport, an electronic record of athletes' blood profiles to assess changes that may indicate possible doping; and encouraged a pre-emptive strike on prospective gene doping. Rather than being directly influenced by the tensions arising from Cold War nationalisms, it is motivated by a perpetual innovation of detection and surveillance techniques justified by the claim that athletes have access to newer, undetectable substances and methods. Moral entrepreneurship is still an important piece of the regime, but it has become institutionalised as moral technopreneurialism. The moral crusade against doping and the drive for innovation go hand in hand. On the one hand, doping and its regulation constitute a tale of medical experts and rule creators leveraging science to accomplish a moral crusade against the impurities of sport. On the other, it is a narrative in which a group of moral entrepreneurs' commitment to innovation serves a performative function that continues the regime and also clouds the social dynamics that enabled the initial condemnation of doping in sport.

The anti-doping story resonates in large part because technological innovation is a compelling actor who has helped to script the current anti-doping regime; however, it comes with consequences. The resulting arms race logic has contributed to shifting attention away from the moral impetus of protecting athletes' health to a more narrow preoccupation with detecting evidence of doping – as a physical impurity presumed to be symbolic of a moral impurity. Anti-doping technologies operate in the service of ideology, though veiling it as the pursuit of a truth-claim. The means of condemning doping in sport exemplify Epstein's point that perceptions of credibility, even scientific credibility, are 'simultaneously an outcome of the competing forces brought to bear in struggles and a marker of the thickening of social ties'.[92] This historical reflection evidences some of those struggles, revealing that the unique character of these processes has since come to embrace a perpetuating cycle in which innovation appears necessary to advance the perception that anti-doping technologies have the capacity to counteract more sophisticated doping athletes. The vilification of doping remains, but the institutional contours instilling it as a morally condemnable offence are distinctly technopreneurial.

Acknowledgements

My sincere thanks to two anonymous reviewers, as this article benefitted significantly from their encouraging and critical feedback. The National Science Foundation Law and Social Science Program (Grant No. SES-0851536) and the International Olympic Committee Postgraduate Grant Programme provided financial support for this research. Her research focuses on the relationships between embodiment, regulation and technoscience and has been funded by the International Olympic Committee, the National Science Foundation, the National Endowment for the Humanities and WADA.

Notes on Contributor

Kathryn Henne is a Research Fellow at the Regulatory Institutions Network, which is housed at the Australian National University. Her research focuses on the relationships between embodiment, regulation and technoscience and has been funded by the International Olympic Committee, the National Science Foundation, the National Endowment for the Humanities and WADA.

Notes

1. Dimeo, *History of Drug Use*, 136.
2. Wrynn, "Human Factor," 211.
3. More detailed analyses include Beamish and Ritchie, *Fastest, Highest, Strongest*; Dimeo, *History of Drug Use*; Hoberman, *Mortal Engines*; Houlihan, *Dying to Win*; and Hunt, *Drug Games.*
4. Park, "Governing Doped Bodies."
5. Goode, *Sport Doping as Deviance*; Henne, *Origins of the International Olympic Committee Medical Commission*, 11; and Stokvis, *Moral Entrepreneurship and Doping Cultures.*
6. Becker, *Outsiders*, 147–8.
7. For other discussions of technopreneurialism, see Kenway et al., *Haunting the Knowledge Economy*, 31–52 and Ong, *Neoliberalism as Exception*, 181–94.
8. Franklin, "Science as Culture, Cultures of Science," 179.
9. Fouché, "Cycling's 'Fix'."
10. Haraway ("Situated Knowledges," 582) refers specifically to the 'god trick' as the presumptive claim that science can have 'infinite vision'. This illusion, she explains, is merely one way of seeing and certainly not an all-knowing way.
11. Hunt, *Drug Games* and Hunt, Dimeo, and Jedlicka, "Historical Roots of Today's Problems."
12. Park, "Governing Doped Bodies."
13. There are noteworthy limitations to relying on these primary texts. There is a 20-year embargo on IOC documents, which, given the time frame of this article, is not significant. There is, however, no guarantee that documents containing contentious, disconcerting or humiliating information about the IOC or its members are available to researchers.
14. Gusfield, *Symbolic Crusade* and Reinarman, "Moral Entrepreneurs and Political Economy."
15. Becker, *Outsiders*, 147.
16. Dimeo, *History of Drug Use*, 95.
17. Hunt, Dimeo, and Jedlicka, "Historical Roots of Today's Problems," 55 and Keys, *Globalising Sport.*
18. Beamish and Ritchie, "From Chivalrous 'Brothers-in-Arms'" and Gleaves, "Doped Professionals and Clean Amateurs."
19. Beamish and Ritchie, "From Chivalrous 'Brothers-in-Arms'," 361–3.
20. Dimeo, *History of Drug Use*, 94–5.

21. Haraway, "Situated Knowledges," 581.
22. Barnes, "Olympic Drug Testing," 23.
23. Ibid.
24. Dirix and Sturbois, *First Thirty Years*.
25. IOC Minutes of the 56th General Session, 9. IOC Archives, Lausanne.
26. Cited in Hunt, *Drug Games*, 10.
27. Ibid., 11.
28. Møller, "Knud Enemark Jensen's Death."
29. Dimeo, Hunt, and Bowers, "Saint or Sinner?" and Hunt, *Drug Games*.
30. For more information about Porritt's tenure, see Hunt, *Drug Games*, 12–23.
31. Porritt, "Doping."
32. Cited in Todd and Todd, "Significant Events in the History of Drug Testing," 68.
33. Beamish and Ritchie, "From Chivalrous 'Brothers-in-Arms'," 361.
34. Hunt, *Drug Games*, 14–5.
35. Cited in Houlihan, *Dying to Win*, 151.
36. IOC, Press Release, September 27, 1967, 2.
37. Dimeo, *History of Drug Use*.
38. La Cava, "Use of Drugs in Competitive Sport," 53.
39. Prokop, "Drug Abuse in International Athletes," 86.
40. Dirix, "Doping Problem at the Tokyo and Mexico City Olympic Games," 185.
41. IOC, Press Release, September 27, 1967.
42. Ibid.
43. Becker, *Outsiders*, 156.
44. See Hoberman, *Testosterone Dreams*. Dimeo, Hunt, and Bowers ("Saint of Sinner?") re-examine these characterizations of de Mérode by considering the circumstances and events surrounding his Chairmanship, a nuanced reading that this study supports.
45. Medical Commission meeting minutes, December 20, 1967, 2. IOC Archives, Lausanne.
46. Ibid., 3.
47. Ibid., 2.
48. Beckett, "Future of the Olympic Movement."
49. Epstein, *Impure Science*, 26.
50. Medical Commission meeting minutes, December 20, 1967, 3. IOC Archives, Lausanne.
51. A. de Mérode, Letter to A. Brundage, September 6, 1968. IOC Archives, Lausanne.
52. Beamish and Ritchie ("From Chivalrous 'Brothers-in-Arms' to the Eligible Athlete") provide a closer reading of how these changes not only affected the rules around Olympic participation but also reconfigured Olympic principles.
53. A. Brundage, Letter to A. de Mérode (copied to International Federations, NOCs and IOC) (underline in original), September 14, 1968. IOC Archives, Lausanne.
54. Medical Commission meeting minutes, July 13–14, 1968, 3. IOC Archives, Lausanne.
55. J. Thiébault, Report on the Medical Commission of the International Olympic Committee on the Grenoble Games, 1969, 12 (translation). IOC Archives, Lausanne.
56. Ibid., 1.
57. Medical Commission meeting minutes, July 13–14, 1968, 4. IOC Archives, Lausanne.
58. Landry and Yerlès, *International Olympic Committee One Hundred Years*, 167, 257.
59. Dimeo, Hunt, and Bowers, "Saint or Sinner?" 933.
60. Ibid.
61. Beamish and Ritchie, *Fastest, Highest, Strongest*.
62. Beamish and Ritchie, "From Chivalrous 'Brothers-in-Arms'," 362–3; Beamish and Ritchie, *Fastest, Highest, Strongest*; and Hoberman, *Mortal Engines*.
63. Woodland, *Dope*, 57.
64. Dimeo, *History of Drug Use*, 79.
65. Hunt, Dimeo, and Jedlicka, "Historical Roots of Today's Problems," 57.
66. NZ Olympic and British Commonwealth Games Association Inc., Letter to Monique Berlioux, March 19, 1973. IOC Archives, Lausanne.
67. Report on the Medical Commission, Sex Testing and Doping, December 13, 1974, 8. IOC Archives, Lausanne.
68. W. Winterbottom, Letter to International Federations, National Governing Bodies of Sport and other interested Organizations, October 30, 1973. IOC Archives, Lausanne.

69. Report on the Medical Commission, Sex Testing and Doping, December 13, 1974, 11. IOC Archives, Lausanne.
70. Dimeo, *History of Drug Use*, 83–6.
71. Ibid., 85.
72. *Track and Field News*, February 1, 1973, enclosure sent by M. Berlioux to A. de Mérode, March 14, 1973. IOC Archives, Lausanne.
73. W. Winterbottom, Letter to International Federations, National Governing Bodies of Sport and other interested Organizations, October 30, 1973. IOC Archives, Lausanne.
74. R. Bannister, Letter to Lord Killanin, November 1, 1973. IOC Archives, Lausanne.
75. Ibid.
76. Historical analyses attest to Western fears focusing on hypermasculinised athletes in women's events (e.g. Beamish and Ritchie, "The Spectre of Steroids").
77. Cited in Landry and Yerlès, *International Olympic Committee One Hundred Years*, 257.
78. Beamish and Ritchie, "From Chivalrous 'Brothers-in-Arms'," 365.
79. "Anabolic Steroids Used in Commonwealth Games," Press Release, May 8, 1974. IOC Archives, Lausanne.
80. Organising Committee of the Games of the XXI Olympiad, Official Report, 454.
81. J. Worrall, Letter to A. de Mérode, January 3, 1975. IOC Archives, Lausanne.
82. Beckett, "Misuse of Drugs in Sports," 190.
83. G. Schödl, Letter to A. de Mérode, August 31, 1976. IOC Archives, Lausanne.
84. Ibid.
85. IOC Medical Commission minutes, October 14–15, 1976, 1; Declaration of the Bulgarian Weightlifting Federation, enclosure sent by Secretary General of Bulgarian NOC, N. Andonov, to the IOC Medical Commission, September 11, 1972. IOC Archives, Lausanne.
86. The cost of testing surpassed 2 million US dollars at the 1976 Montreal Games (Al-Habet, Redda, and Lee, "Uses and Abuses of Anabolic Steroids," 221).
87. Dimeo, Hunt, and Bowers, "Saint or Sinner?," 934.
88. "Olympic Athletes Cleared," (*Washington Post*, February 25, 1980).
89. IOC Medical Commission, "Doping Control at Games of the XXIInd Olympiad," February 1981.
90. Cited in Dimeo, Hunt, and Bowers, "Saint or Sinner?," 935.
91. Landry and Yerlès, *International Olympic Committee One Hundred Years*.
92. Epstein, *Impure Science*, 26.

References

Al-Habet, S., K. Redda, and H. Lee. "Uses and Abuses of Anabolic Steroids by Athletes." In *Cocaine, Marijuana, Designer Drugs: Chemistry, Pharmacology, and Behaviour*, edited by K. Redda, C. Walker and G. Barnett, 211–232. Boca Raton, FL: CRC Press, 1989.

Barnes, L. "Olympic Drug Testing: Improvements without Progress." *The Physician and Sports Medicine* 8, no. 6 (1980): 21–24.

Beamish, R., and I. Ritchie. *Fastest, Highest, Strongest: A Critique of High Performance Sport*. New York: Routledge, 2006.

Beamish, R., and I. Ritchie. "From Chivalrous 'Brothers-in-Arms' to the Eligible Athlete: Changed Principles and the IOC's Banned Substance List." *International Review for the Sociology of Sport* 39, no. 4 (2004): 355–371.

Beamish, R., and I. Ritchie. "The Spectre of Steroids: Nazi Propaganda, Cold War Anxiety and Patriarchal Paternalism." *International Journal of the History of Sport* 22, no. 5 (2005): 777–795.

Becker, H. *Outsiders: Studies in Sociology of Deviance*. New York: Free Press, 1963.

Beckett, A. "The Future of the Olympic Movement." In *Drug Controversy in Sport: The Socio-ethical and Medical Issues*, edited by R. Laura and S. White, 25–37. Sydney: Allen and Unwin, 1991.

Beckett, A. "Misuse of Drugs in Sports." *British Journal of Sports Medicine* 12 (1979): 185–194.

Dimeo, P. *A History of Drug Use in Sport 1876–1976: Beyond Good and Evil*. London: Routledge, 2007.

Dimeo, P., T. Hunt, and M. T. Bowers. "Saint or Sinner?: A Reconsideration of the Career of Alexandre de Mérode, Chair of the International Olympic Committee's Medical Commission, 1967–2002." *The International Journal of the History of Sport* 28, no. 6 (2011): 925–940.

Dirix, A. "The Doping Problem at the Tokyo and Mexico City Olympic Games." *Journal of Sports Medicine and Fitness* 6 (1963): 183–186.

Dirix, A., and X. Sturbois. *The First Thirty Years of the International Olympic Committee Medical Commission 1967–1997*. Lausanne: International Olympic Committee (IOC Booklet Series, "History and Facts"), 1998.

Epstein, S. *Impure Science: AIDS, Activism, and the Politics of Knowledge*. Berkeley: University of California Press, 1996.

Fouché, R. "Cycling's 'Fix'." *Journal of Sport & Social Issues* 33, no. 1 (2006): 97–99.

Franklin, S. "Science as Culture, Cultures of Science." *Annual Review of Anthropology* 24 (1995): 163–184.

Gleaves, J. "Doped Professionals and Clean Amateurs: Amateurism's Influence on the Modern Philosophy of Anti-Doping." *Journal of Sport History* 38, no. 2 (2011): 237–254.

Goode, E. *Sport Doping as Deviance: Anti-Doping as Moral Panic*. Norderstedt: Books on Demand GmbH, 2011.

Gusfield, J. *Symbolic Crusade: Status Politics and the American Temperance Movement*. Urbana: University of Illinois Press, 1963.

Haraway, D. "Situated Knowledges: The Science Question in Feminism and the Privilege of Partial Knowledge." *Feminist Studies* 14, no. 3 (1988): 575–599.

Henne, K. *The Origins of the International Olympic Committee Medical Commission and Its Technocratic Regime: An Historiographic Investigation of Anti-Doping Regulation*. Lausanne: International Olympic Committee, 2010. http://doc.rero.ch/record/17372

Hoberman, J. *Mortal Engines: The Science of Performance and the Dehumanisation of Sport*. New York: The Free Press, 1992.

Hoberman, J. *Testosterone Dreams: Rejuvenation, Aphrodisia, Doping*. Berkeley: University of California Press, 2006.

Houlihan, B. *Dying to Win: Doping in Sport and the Development of Anti-Doping Policy*. 2nd ed. Strasbourg: Council of Europe, 2002.

Hunt, T. *Drug Games: The International Olympic Committee and the Politics of Doping, 1960–2008*. Austin: University of Texas Press, 2011.

Hunt, T., P. Dimeo, and S. R. Jedlicka. "The Historical Roots of Today's Problems: A Critical Appraisal of the International Anti-Doping Movement." *Performance Enhancement & Health* 1 (2012): 55–60.

Kenway, J., E. Bullen, J. Fahey, and S. Robb. *Haunting the Knowledge Economy*. New York: Routledge, 2006.

Keys, B. J. *Globalising Sport: National Rivalry and International Community in the 1930s*. Cambridge, MA: Harvard University Press, 2006.

La Cava, G. "The Use of Drugs in Competitive Sport." *Bulletin du Comité International Olympique* 78 (1962): 52–53.

Landry, F., and M. Yerlès. *The International Olympic Committee One Hundred Years: The Idea – The Presidents – The Achievements*. Lausanne: The International Olympic Committee, 1996.

Møller, V. "Knud Enemark Jensen's Death During the 1960 Rome Olympics: A Search for Truth?" *Sport in History* 25, no. 3 (2009): 452–471.

Ong, A. *Neoliberalism as Exception: Mutations in Citizenship and Sovereignty*. Durham, NC: Duke University Press, 2006.

Park, J. "Governing Doped Bodies: The World Anti-Doping Agency and the Global Culture of Surveillance." *Cultural Studies ↔ Critical Methodologies* 5, no. 2 (2005): 174–186.

Porritt, A. "Doping." *The Journal of Sports Medicine and Physical Fitness* 5, no. 3 (1965): 166–168.

Prokop, L. "Drug Abuse in International Athletes." *Journal of Sport Medicine* 3, no. 2 (1975): 85–87.

Reinarman, C. "Moral Entrepreneurs and Political Economy: Historical and Ethnographic Notes on the Construction of the Cocaine Menace." *Contemporary Crises* 3, no. 3 (1979): 225–254.

Stokvis, R. *Moral Entrepreneurship and Doping Cultures in Sport*. ASSR Working Paper Series, Amsterdam: Amsterdam School for Social Science Research (2003): 1–25.

Todd, J., and T. Todd. "Significant Events in the History of Drug Testing and the Olympic Movement." In *Doping in Elite Sport: The Politics of Drugs in the Olympic Movement*, edited by W. Wilson and W. Derse, 65–128. Champaign, IL: Human Kinetics, 2001.

Woodland, L. *Dope: The Use of Drugs in Sport*. London: David & Charles, 1980.

Wrynn, A. "The Human Factor: Science, Medicine and the International Olympic Committee, 1900–70." *Sport in Society* 7, no. 2 (2004): 211–231.

Drugs, the Law, and the Downfall of Dancer's Image at the 1968 Kentucky Derby: A Case Study on Human Conceptions of Domesticated Animals

Thomas M. Hunt, Scott R. Jedlicka and Matthew T. Bowers

Department of Kinesiology and Health Education, University of Texas at Austin, Austin, TX, USA

The disqualification of Dancer's Image at the 1968 Kentucky Derby for the presence of a prohibited substance reveals much about the human–animal relationship. The horse was, on the one hand, depicted in anthropomorphic terms as an honourable competitor unjustly stripped of a victory. At the same time, Dancer's Image was treated as simply a piece of physical property. In short, human conceptions of domesticated animals are dichotomous in nature.

At 4:40 p.m. on Saturday, May 4, 1968, 14 thoroughbred horses leapt from the starting gates of the Churchill Downs racetrack, signalling the start of the 94th Kentucky Derby. For most of the first mile, a beautiful grey colt named Dancer's Image remained at the back of the pack. As 100,000 spectators in the grandstands and a television audience of 18 million watched, the colt made a move along the rail in the last quarter-mile. The horse's jockey, Bobby Ussery, having lost his whip somewhere along the way, furiously urged greater and greater speed until Dancer's Image emerged from the pack at the eighth pole and then crossed the finished wire, victorious, with a length-and-a-half lead. Having won $122,600 in one of the sporting world's greatest extravaganzas, Peter Fuller, the colt's exultant owner, exclaimed at a post-race party amidst toasts of champagne, 'I wasn't exactly wrong when I said we had come to win, was I?'[1]

On the Monday morning following the race, however, Fuller received a cryptic phone call from a friend staying at Louisville's Brown Hotel. 'They've got a problem with your horse's [drug] test', claimed the caller. 'It's very serious'.[2] Later that day, the Stewards of the Kentucky Derby announced that Dancer's Image had been disqualified after a urinalysis detected Phenylbutazone (trade name Butazolidin), a non-steroidal anti-inflammatory drug prohibited by rule 14.06 of the Rules of Racing and the Kentucky State Racing Act, in the horse's system. 'The words staggered me', said Lou Cavalaris, who, as the horse's trainer, was subsequently suspended. 'I was spellbound. I just stood there. I've been in this game 21 years and I've never done anything wrong.'[3] The *Chicago Tribune* declared in reference to the event that 'the sport of horse racing in this country was rocked by the worst scandal in its 300-year history'.[4]

The episode, which was the first and only instance in which a horse was disqualified from a Kentucky Derby due to the presence of an illegal substance, also made the cover of

Sports Illustrated magazine, in whose pages it was declared 'the year's major sports story'.[5] A legal battle ensued soon thereafter, culminating in a 1972 decision by the Court of Appeals of Kentucky, which influenced the later direction of drug controls in American horse racing.[6] The mysterious nature of the battle, marked by the involvement of a shadowy veterinarian and accusations by Fuller of a conspiracy against his horse, led Court of Appeals Judge Catinna to write, 'There are numerous contradictions and even contradictions of contradictions throughout this entire record.'[7] It was, to borrow from Winston Churchill's famous turn of phrase, 'a riddle wrapped in a mystery inside an enigma'.[8]

While the cultural dynamics at play in the use of drugs by human competitors has received detailed scholarly attention in recent years, far less has been written about the issue from an equine perspective.[9] This discrepancy, at least in part, derives from the fact that historians (including, with a few noteworthy exceptions, those who have studies sport) have traditionally neglected issues relating to non-human actors.[10] To be fair, the fact that animals do not produce written records presents a significant obstacle to those interested in conducting such research. While innovative scholars have in recent years begun to identify methodological solutions to this dilemma, a number of matters pertaining to the place of domesticated actors in society deserve further consideration. Of these, perhaps the most significant concerns the nature of human conceptions regarding their non-human counterparts.[11]

Historical scrutiny of equestrian sport possesses considerable potential to advance our understanding of these conceptions.[12] Under statutory law and judicial precedent, domesticated animals are categorised as property; much as slaves did prior to abolition, animals under this framework each possess a certain monetary value determined by market forces.[13] As property, domesticated animals exist in a situation in which human owners exercise command over their living conditions. This is the case, for example, regarding the medical treatments and food ingested by thoroughbred horses that race in athletic competitions. There is something to be said for this distribution of authority; humans are, after all, well equipped to distinguish between healthy meals and unhealthy ones. For horses, on the other hand, and as a popular comedian once joked, 'It's all the same oat-bag'.[14]

Even so, the fact that human actors maintain power over that oat-bag suggests something important about the position of domesticated animals in the social order; they are, in a very real sense, physical assets that are owned and controlled. It would be a mistake, however, to characterise the relationship between humans and their non-human counterparts solely in such terms. Indeed, a large part of humanity sees domesticated animals as possessing an emotional importance that deserves protection.[15] The title of a recent editorial on the website of the digital fan community Horse Racing Nation even went so far as to declare from this perspective that 'Horses are people too'.[16]

In the historical records pertaining to the 1968 Kentucky Derby, one can find a number of similarly anthropomorphic modes of description. In these, Dancer's Image is depicted as the possessor of a human-like moral code centred on the noble pursuit of athletic victory. When stripped of his victory, Dancer's Image is shown in these representations as suffering a tremendous emotional blow. Alongside such instances of anthropomorphism, however, one can also find numerous cases in which the horse's disqualification is discussed in purely monetary terms. Given its ability to shed light on these seemingly contradictory patterns of belief, the 1968 Kentucky Derby provides a useful case study through which to examine the relationship between humans and domesticated animals.

Regulatory Debates on Anti-inflammatory Drugs in Equestrian Sport

The years leading up to the 1968 Kentucky Derby featured a number of debates on the administration of drugs to performance horses. A 1960 *Sports Illustrated* article on the use of Butazolidin provides a useful example as to how the matter was discussed from a property perspective.[17] In that article, California owner Rex Ellsworth was paraphrased as saying that 'he would not stand a horse at stud whose record was tainted with Butazolidin victories'. As for what the drug might mean for the financial position of the broader racing industry, a general consensus existed among those interviewed for the article that the drug constituted a worrisome threat. Calumet Farm's legendary Jimmy Jones contended, for example, that 'No matter what you call a medication, in the public mind it's [*sic*] dope. Well, it has taken horse racing a long time to build up the public's confidence, and it shouldn't do anything to lose that confidence.'[18]

In arguing for the enactment of stricter controls on anti-inflammatory medications, some members of the racing establishment also cited a moral duty on the part of humanity to protect the lesser creatures of the earth. Among those to do so was Keene Daingerfield, then president of the Society of North American Racing Officials. 'People keep telling me that Sandy Koufax [a famous baseball player] used Butazolidin every time he pitched', he said, 'But Koufax knew what he was doing. ... The horse doesn't have this option.'[19] In a passage on the need for a rule prohibiting the administration of drugs at any point during the 48 hours prior to a race, a 1959 report issued by the National Association of Racing Commissions featured a similarly anthropomorphic claim:

> In a relatively short span of years, we have seen horses make a transition from being raced for a few days or weeks each year at local tracks and fairs to year around racing with flying trips to distant points considered commonplace. The large increases in purse values are further inducements to run horses as often as possible, wherever possible. It is therefore reasonable to assume that some horses may be subject to the tensions that afflict busy humans and require the use of vitamins, sedatives, and tranquillizers.
>
> With such general use of medicines, hormones, vitamins, and food supplements, including some drugs of questionable legality and some which cannot be detected by the racing chemists, the 48-hour rule governing medication seems to be more needed today than ever before.[20]

In terms of the dichotomous attitudes of humans towards domesticated animals, it should also be noted that the opponents to the regulation of anti-inflammatory mediations based their countervailing arguments on the same grounds of property and ethical duty.[21] In terms of the former, Kentucky horse breeder Bull Hancock declared that 'he [did] not believe the drug's contribution to a horse's record would detract from his value as a stud'.[22] Jim Fitzsimmons, a Hall of Fame trainer and the first president of the Horsemen's Benevolent and Protective Association, asserted, for example, that 'if you're going to protect the public, you should be allowed to send horses out in the best condition possible'.[23] Ralph Choisser, steward of the Illinois Racing Board agreed. 'Today's tracks are much harder than they used to be and horses get "sored" up', he said, 'I believe that in the long run Butazolidin may make for more formful [*sic*] racing'.[24]

In the end, some states took lenient positions on the use of anti-inflammatory drugs while others adopted strict controls.[25] The resulting regulatory inconsistency, in which horses could benefit from drugs like Butazolidin at some tracks but not at others, was perhaps best illustrated in a statement overheard after a horse named Carry Black failed to win the Triple Crown by losing the 1961 Belmont Stakes in New York. 'That just shows what that stuff can do', a reporter recalled hearing, 'They could use of [*sic*] butazolidin in Maryland, where he won the Preakness, and in Kentucky, where he won the Derby, but not here in New York'.[26] As the decade rolled on, however, the balance of opinion shifted in clear favour of stricter controls on anti-inflammatory medications. Though it was one of the last states to do so, the state of Kentucky in the end went along with this line of judgment and banned the race-time usage of Butazolidin.[27]

It was in this context that, shortly after his appearance at the Churchill Downs winner's circle, Dancer's Image was taken to a set of stables known as the 'detention barn' where a sample of his saliva was taken. Approximately an hour-and-a-half later, a urine sample was obtained by Veterinarian George Dickinson while Cavalaris's assistant trainer Robert Barnard watched.[28] The specimen, anonymously tagged number 3956U, was taken to an adjacent trailer owned by the Louisville Testing Laboratory, Inc., the official chemist for the Kentucky State Racing Commission. Five chemical tests were then performed that each indicated the presence of Butazolidin. A hearing was subsequently held on May 13, 14 and 15 by the Stewards of the Churchill Downs racetrack, who concluded that the drug was indeed present. They, in addition, decreed that the purse should be redistributed, but that bets and the payment of pari-mutuel tickets would not be affected.[29] Remarkably, only one other horse from the race – the fifth-place Kentucky Sherry – had its saliva and urine sampled; Forward Pass, later declared the winner, was never tested.[30] Dancer's Image therefore became, in Fuller's words, 'the only horse that ever won the race on Saturday and lost it on Monday'.[31]

Dichotomous Representations in the Legal Proceedings Concerning Dancer's Image

Fuller believed that a mistake must surely have been made in the disqualification of Dancer's Image and so he filed an appeal with the Kentucky State Racing Commission. 'If one of my people said that we did use the drug', Fuller asserted, 'we wouldn't have contested. We felt that obviously it didn't happen as far as we are concerned.' Speaking to the media, he emphasised again that 'I know that I did nothing wrong, and I know that no members of my organization did anything wrong'.[32] The stakes for Fuller in the appeal's outcome were high. In addition to the revocation of the Kentucky Derby's monetary prize, he as the owner of Dancer's Image faced the loss of millions of dollars in stud fees.[33] The property value of Dancer's Image would, of course, also plummet. Lloyds of London had already reduced its insurance valuation of Dancer's Image in the aftermath of its failed drug test from $1.5 to $1 million.[34] Outlining his fears, Fuller stated that '"everything is waiting on this hearing". Commercial breeders say something to the effect that "I'll see you later". ... They want to know – is this a real horse, or is this a horse that has to be helped [by illegal drugs].'[35]

Fuller consistently also discussed the case in anthropomorphic terms, however. In testifying before the racing commission, he said, for instance:

> [W]hen you have raised the horse yourself, and you have bred him and you have watched him grow and you have admittedly made mistakes with him, and you have good things with him and you have all the experience with the horse, then its [the positive test] a very real thing ...
>
> This horse is no phony horse, this horse didn't win races with mirrors [*sic*]. This horse won races on his ability, not with the help of anything except the ability he had.
>
> I have to clear my horse's name.[36]

As the horse's trainer, Cavalaris made a similar claim of emotional connection. 'I'm innocent and so are my men', he said. 'They love Dancer's Image, just as I do'.[37] Just as countless people do regarding the pets that inhabit their homes, Fuller and Cavalaris perceived Dancer's Image as a beloved family member – and one with a sense of personal reputation that deserved protection.[38]

Fuller's feelings along these lines could not entirely transcend his sense of the horse as a piece of property, however. In a 1985 interview, Fuller began with an emotional statement that 'It took a while for the hurt to fade [from the disqualification], but to be honest, I felt really badly for the horse'. This assertion was followed, though, with a bitter grievance as to the financial losses he suffered in the episode. 'In the pedigree records [which affect the monetary value of horses]', he complained, 'in the United States, unlike in Europe and Japan, the disqualification is not written in. It's never even mentioned that he won.'[39]

Those without close personal connection to Dancer's Image adopted in the immediate aftermath of the race attitudes based almost entirely on this legal paradigm in which performance horses were categorised as property. Indeed, the unprecedented degree of national interest in the case sparked worries in the Kentucky racing industry about the result's potential effects on the state economy. A 1968 survey that was jointly sponsored by the Thoroughbred Breeders of Kentucky, the Kentucky State Racing Commission and the Horsemen's Benevolent Protective Association showed the extent of the state's dependence on the industry. The study estimated that thoroughbred racing attracted some 500,000 visitors to the Lexington area alone and that approximately $250 million was invested into one aspect or another of the state's horse industry. Of more immediate concern, the study found that more than $4.1 million in pari-mutuel and admission taxes had been paid into the Kentucky Treasury in 1968 alone.[40] It was therefore noted that the gamblers who paid those taxes were interested in the Commission's deliberations given that their members had bet a record $2,350,470 on the 1968 Derby.[41] The disqualification of Dancer's Image, in other words, represented a great deal of money to a great number of people; the fact that those individuals saw the horse in purely property terms should thus not at all surprise.

Meeting at the Kentucky Fair and Exposition Center during the last two months of the year, the state's five racing commissioners began their hearings on the race. In his opening statement, Fuller's lawyer, Arthur Grafton, acknowledged that 'chemical procedures for the detection and the identification of the many drugs which may be given to a race horse are obviously complicated and difficult'. And so, he continued, 'everyone knows that a chemist is not infallible, being an ordinary human being like the rest of us'. The Commission's official chemist, Kenneth Smith, according to Grafton used tests that 'were grossly inadequate for the purpose of proving the presence of the drug [Butazolidin], even if each of the tests had been adequately and properly conducted'.[42] This focus on the appropriateness of the laboratory analyses redirected the debate away from media speculation that some sort of conspiracy was at play. As for the Derby's point of view, State Attorney General George Rabe responded that 'the evidence on the whole in this case that will be presented by us will show the presence of phenylbutazone and/or a derivative thereof in the urine of the horse'.[43] After 14 days worth of hearings, the Commission issued an order that sustained the prior decision by the Stewards of the Churchill Downs to disallow Fuller's victory.

Appealing to yet a higher authority, this time the Franklin, Kentucky, Circuit Court, Fuller alleged that the Commission had denied him the due process of law by rendering a decision without substantial supportive evidence.[44] In terms of the human–animal relationship, the appeal represented yet another example of the legal and emotional dynamics of human attitudes towards non-human actors. On the one hand, Fuller recalled with tears in his eyes--and in anthropomorphic terms--that 'I would like them to remember Dancer [Dancer's Image] as a guy that made a stretch run. Certainly his owner and his pals will never forget.'[45] The appeal, in his words, was therefore 'a matter of principle ... a matter of the horse's record. He won the record. He won the race.'[46] But the legal reality was that such anthropomorphic references mattered little. Fuller could only appeal based on the notion that his property interests as a human owner had been taken away without due process of law.

Having found that property-based argument compelling, Circuit Judge Henry Meigs reinstated Dancer's Image as the rightful champion of the Derby. After objecting to Judge Meigs's order that the 1968 Derby purse be redistributed and that they should repay Fuller for his legal expenses, the members of the state racing commission responded with an appeal of their own to the Kentucky Court of Appeals.[47] California's controversial decision around this time to legalise the use of Butazolidin in its races underscored the importance of the case to the national racing establishment. Leonard Foote, chief investigator of the California racing board, claimed that 'we do not permit drugging. Butazolidin is in no way a stimulant.'[48] The resulting contradictory nature of drug controls in thoroughbred racing caused horse owners and trainers in Illinois to consider boycotting races within their state.[49] In addition, British racing officials, worried as a result of the Fuller lawsuit about legal complications at their own races, halted enforcement of their own drug rules.[50] The extent to which such legal battles as Fuller's were influencing the direction of the athletics world even caused one *Washington Post* columnist to lament:

> The periwigs and perukes [*sic*] of law are taking over in sports and the uniform of the day seems to be the black roe [*sic*] of the presiding justice. ... The legal battles have only just begun[, however]. You can't tell your sports without a law degree these days.[51]

In the next step of the judicial process, Rabe filed a brief for the Court of Appeals on July 30, 1971, in which he asserted the gist of the Kentucky Racing Commission's argument. 'The Franklin Circuit Court', he wrote, 'proceeded to make its own finding, ignoring both those of the commission and the evidence to support them.'[52] The crux of the matter thus turned on two interrelated issues: first, the commission's authority to promulgate rules and regulations regarding the use of drugs in its races, and second, on the accuracy of its testing procedures. Writing for the Court of Appeals, Judge Catinna asserted that 'the Commission was vested with all powers necessary and proper to carry out fully and effectively those duties imposed upon it by the statutes', which included rulemaking authority for preventing 'the administration of drugs ... for the purpose of affecting the speed or health of horses in races'. Moreover, 'The commission as the trier of the facts saw each witness and was in a superior position to evaluate the situation as well as the conduct and demeanor of each witness as he testified.' Most importantly, Catinna wrote, 'All witnesses agreed that a positive result on the five tests given by Smith would be sufficient to support a positive finding.'[53]

In accordance with these findings, the Court of Appeals ordered that the earlier decision by the Kentucky State Racing Commission be reinstated and that Forward Pass be declared the winner. Fuller was again dismayed and stated that he was 'stunned by the decision. I thought the matter had already been settled.' His economic losses were staggering. In addition to his legal expenses, Fuller claimed that the court battle had prevented him from recovering a tremendous amount in stud fees.[54] The owner later sadly concluded, 'I felt I was entitled to both the trophy and the money. This ruling, however, seems to me to be directly contrary to the law'.[55]

Conclusion

By demonstrating the legal and emotional dynamics at play on the subject, the historical record of the 1968 Kentucky Derby helps to shed light on the human–animal relationship. The many anthropomorphic depictions of the event as an injustice to an honourable competitor reflected, on the one side, a powerful set of human beliefs regarding the emotional value of domesticated animals. Others that focused on the financial implications of the episode for Fuller did so under a countervailing, and equally real legal paradigm that treats domesticated animals as physical property. The fact that Dancer's Image was often simultaneously referred to as both an emotional being and as a piece of property says much about the complicated nature of human attitudes towards non-human actors.

Notes on Contributors

Thomas M. Hunt, J.D., Ph.D., is Assistant Professor in the Department of Kinesiology and Health Education at The University of Texas at Austin, where he also holds an appointment as Assistant Director for Academic Affairs at the H.J. Lutcher Stark Center for Physical Culture and Sports.

Scott R. Jedlicka is a doctoral candidate in sport management at the University of Texas at Austin. His research focuses on sport and international relations.

Matthew T. Bowers, Ph.D., is Clinical Assistant Professor in the Department of Kinesiology and Health Education at The University of Texas at Austin, where his research explores youth sport development.

Notes

1. This narrative is based largely on Tower, "And the Last was First." In addition, a video of the race is available online by the Kentucky Derby. It provides the announcer's description of Dancer's Image 'coming like a house a'fire'; available at: http://www.kentuckyderby.com/history/year/1968 (accessed January, 28 2013). The money won by Fuller is found on the 1968 'Kentucky Derby Media Guide Chart', which is also available online by the Kentucky Derby at: http://www.kentuckyderby.com/sites/kentuckyderby.com/files/charts/1968.pdf (accessed January 28, 2013). Though written for a popular rather than academic audience, Toby's *Dancer's Image* provides a useful narrative of the race and its aftermath. A book for children on the event has also been published: Labrie, *Dancer's Image*.
2. The phone call was from Walter Jones. Quoted in McEvoy, *Great Horse Racing Mysteries*, 112.
3. Cavalaris quoted in Tower, "It Was a Bitter Pill."
4. Rivera, "Vet Hits Handling."
5. Tower, "It was a Bitter Pill". The drug protocols in place at the 1968 Kentucky Derby are usefully discussed in Novak, "The Derby Drug."
6. Kentucky State Racing Commission v. Peter Fuller, 481 S.W.2d 298 (1972).
7. Judge Catinna, Ibid., 307. A journalist account of the controversy surrounding the 1968 Kentucky Derby can be found in McEvoy, *Great Horse Racing Mysteries*, 98–126. For its legal complexities, begin with Toby, *Dancer's Image*.
8. Churchill's comment was made in a 1939 speech. A draft of his speech notes is available online by Cambridge University, Churchill College, Online Exhibit: Churchill and Russia: http://www.chu.cam.ac.uk/archives/gallery/Russia/CHAR_09_138_46.php (accessed January 28, 2013).
9. Significant book-length studies published on human doping include Beamish, *Steroids*; Beamish and Ritchie, *Fastest, Highest, Strongest*; Dimeo, *A History of Drug Use*; Hoberman, *Mortal Engines*; Hoberman, *Testosterone Dreams*; Hunt, *Drug Games*; Möller, *The Ethics of Doping*; Möller, *The Scapegoat*; and Waddington, *Sport, Health, and Drugs*. For an early, particularly influential article, see Todd, "Anabolic Steroids." Equestrian doping, it should be

mentioned, is featured in a chapter (pp. 269–90) of Hoberman, *Testosterone Dreams*; and in sections of Cassidy, *Horse People*; Huggins, "Flat Racing"; Huggins, *Horseracing and the British*; and Vamplew, "Sporting Innovation." A notable exception to the absence of historical scholarship on equine doping can also be found in Gleaves, "Enhancing the Odds." For a useful legal article that covers much historical ground on the issue of doping in horseracing, see Friedman, "Oats, Water, Hay." For a general overview of doping in equine sport, consult Tobin, *Drugs and the Performance Horse*. On the ancient roots of equine doping, consult Higgins, "From Ancient Greece." See, for the treatment of a recent case, Squires, *Headless Horsemen*.

10. The traditional neglect of non-human actors has in recent years begun to erode. See, for a brief overview of the study of animals by historians, Ritvo, "History and Animal Studies." For broader introductions to the subject, consult Brants, *Beastly Natures*; and DeMello, *Animals and Society*. For interesting book-length works in the field of 'animal studies', see Anderson, *Creatures of Empire*; Landry *Noble Brutes*; Nelson, *Heart and Blood*; Ritvo, *The Animal Estate*; Rothfels, *Representing Animals*; and Tuan, *Dominance and Affection*. For historical studies that touch on equine sport, see Burnett, "The Sites and Landscapes"; Huggins, "Mingled Pleasure and Speculation"; Huggins, "The Proto-globalisation"; Kay, "Still Going"; Vamplew, *The Turf*; and Vamplew, "Unsporting Behavior." For useful sociological studies pertaining to equine sport, consult Gilbert and Gillett, "Equine Athletes"; and Hedenborg and White, "Changes and Variations." See, for a broad regulatory history of thoroughbred racing, Howland, "Let's Not Spit."
11. For useful discussions of animal agency, see Hribal, "Animals, Agency, and Class"; McFarl, Hediger, and McFarland, "Animals and Agency"; and Steward, "Animal Agency."
12. For a potential model for conducting such research, one might consult Madden, "Imaging the Greyhound"; and McManus and Montoya, "Toward New Understandings."
13. See Francione, "Animals as Property"; Francione, *Animals, Property, and the Law*; and Hauser, Cushman, and Kamen, *People, Property, or Pets?*
14. Seinfeld, "Horses."
15. An interesting historical comparison of the emotional value placed on domesticated animals is provided in Scott, "Death to Poochy." For useful analyses of how changing attitudes might affect how animals are treated under the law in the future, see Hankin, "Not a Living Room Sofa"; Kelch, "Toward a Non-property Status"; and Root, "Man's Best Friend." As for how the increasing emotional value placed on domesticated animals might affect veterinary treatments in the future, consult Nunalee and Weedon, "Modern Trends."
16. "Horses Are People Too," Horse Racing Nation, June 25, 2012, available online at: http://www.horseracingnation.com/news/Horses_are_people_too_123. Dogs possess an even closer emotional connection to humans than horses. See "Are dogs people too?" *Economist*, February 26, 2005, 79.
17. Leggett, "The Mysterious Buty Treatment."
18. Quotes from Ibid., 17.
19. Daingerfield quoted in Plattner, "History of the National HBPA."
20. Report quoted in Addis-Smith, "The Changing Pattern,", 125–6.
21. See, for example, "Race Officials Argue Use of 'Wonder' Drug," *Los Angeles Times*, May 17, 1960. For an attempt during this era to distinguish between ethical and unethical usage of drugs in horse racing, see Berriman, "The Ethical Use." See, for a later such effort, Clarke and Moss, "Veterinary Aspects of Doping."
22. Quoted in Leggett, "The Mysterious Buty Treatment," 17.
23. Fitzsimmons quoted in Plattner, "History of the National HBPA."
24. Choisser quoted in Leggett, "The Mysterious Buty Treatment."
25. This regulatory inconsistency extends beyond anti-inflammatory medications. And it remains an issue today. For calls to unify the regulatory system in horse racing see Breslin, "Reclaiming the Glory"; Frederick, "Saving Silent Sufferers"; and Kluesner, "And They're Off." For a countervailing argument regarding the need to unify the regulatory system, consult Bonnie, "Corrupt Horse Racing Practices Act."
26. Quoted in Haight, "Horses and People."
27. Toby, *Dancer's Image*, 38–9.
28. Tower, "It Was a Bitter Pill."
29. Kentucky State Racing Commission v. Peter Fuller, 299–300.

30. See Tower, "It Was a Bitter Pill".
31. Fuller quoted from Peter Fuller Interview by Jim Bolus, November 17, 1987, Jim Bolus Collection, Kentucky Derby Museum, Louisville Kentucky (hereafter Bolus Collection).
32. Kentucky State Racing Commission Press Release, November 18, 1968, Bolus Collection.
33. Fuller had been offered $1 million for Dancer's Image before the 1968 Derby and the colt had been syndicated for an addition $2 million. Kentucky State Racing Commission Press Release, November 18, 1968, Bolus Collection.
34. Kentucky State Racing Commission Press Release, November 19, 1968, Bolus Collection.
35. Kentucky State Racing Commission Press Release, November 18, 1968, Bolus Collection.
36. Fuller quoted in Toby, *Dancer's Image*, 73.
37. Cavalaris quoted in Toby, *Dancer's Image*, 63.
38. Cavalaris experience is especially instructive on the dichotomous nature of human attitudes towards performance animals. As Dancer's Image's trainer, he held an ethical duty to 'take responsibility' for the horse. This duty arose in the horseracing industry consequent to a mixture of anthropomorphic and financial reasons. On the responsibilities of horse trainers, consult Liebman, "The Trainer Responsibility."
39. Fuller quoted in United Press International. "Peter Fuller's Sentimental Journey: Dancer's Image Owner Will Return to Churchill Downs", *Los Angeles Times*, March 31, 1985.
40. Kentucky State Racing Press Release, November 19, 1968, Bolus Collection.
41. See "Why Derby Penalty Was Held Up", *Chicago Tribune*, May 8, 1968.
42. Kentucky State Racing Commission, Hearing before the Kentucky State Racing Commission re: Appeal of Peter Fuller: Opening Statements of Mr Arthur Grafton and Honourable George F. Rabe, November 18 1968, 2, 4, 6, Bolus Collection.
43. Ibid., 39.
44. Kentucky State Racing Commission v. Peter Fuller, 300.
45. Fuller quote from Fuller interview by Bolus, November 17, 1987, Bolus Collection.
46. Fuller quoted in "Fuller: Appeal was Matter of Principle", *Chicago Tribune*, December 12, 1970.
47. "Decision on Dancer's Image Formally Entered in Court", *New York Times*, January 1, 1971.
48. Becker, "Butazolidin Gives a Lift."
49. Milbert, "Turf Storm," "Boycott Off."
50. See on this point, Brown, "French Keep Pace."
51. Addie, "Sports Having Day."
52. Rabe quoted in "1968 Derby Drug Case Comes to Court Again", *Washington Post*, July 31, 1971.
53. Kentucky State Racing Commission v. Peter Fuller, 300, 307, 304.
54. 'The people that own the better mares haven't really patronized him [Dancer's Image] because of this question', lamented Fuller. This quote of Fuller is from "Court Deprives Dancer's Image of '68 Derby Purse", *New York Times*, April 29, 1972.
55. Fuller quoted in "'68 Derby is Given to Forward Pass", *New York Times*, October 28, 1972.

References

Addie, Bob. 1971. "Sports Having Day in Court." *Washington Post*, September 22.

Addis-Smith, L. F. "The Changing Pattern of 'Doping' in Horse Racing and Its Control." *New Zealand Veterinary Journal* 9, no. 6 (1961): 121–128.

Anderson, Virginia De John. *Creatures of Empire: How Domestic Animals Transformed Early America*. New York: Oxford University Press, 2004.

Beamish, Rob. *Steroids: A New Look at Performance-Enhancing Drugs*. Santa Barbara, CA: Praeger, 2011.

Beamish, Rob, and Ian Ritchie. *Fastest, Highest, Strongest: A Critique of High Performance Sport*. New York: Routledge, 2006.

Becker, Bill. 1971. "Butazolidin Gives a Lift to Santa Anita Favorites." *New York Times*, January 29.

Berriman, J. A. "The Ethical Use of Drugs in Racehorses." *Australian Veterinary Journal* 38, no. 4 (1962): 248–252.

Bonnie, Edward S. "Corrupt Horse Racing Practices Act of 1980: A Threat to State Control of Horse Racing." *Kentucky Law Journal* 70 (1981): 1159–1179.

Brants, Dorothee, ed. *Beastly Natures: Animals, Humans, and the Study of History*. Charlottesville: University of Virginia Press, 2010.

Breslin, Luke P. "Reclaiming the Glory in the 'Sport of Kings' – Uniformity is the Answer." *Seton Hall Journal of Sports and Entertainment Law* 20 (2010): 297–332.

Brown, James. 1971. "French Keep Pace with Horse-Druggers." *New York Times*, August 1.

Burnett, John. "The Sites and Landscapes of Horse Racing in Scotland Before 1860." *Sports Historian* 18, no. 1 (1998): 55–75.

Cassidy, Rebecca Louise. *Horse People: Thoroughbred Culture in Lexington and Newmarket*. Baltimore: Johns Hopkins University Press, 2007.

Clarke, E. G. C., and M. S. Moss. "Veterinary Aspects of Doping." *Equine Veterinary Journal* 9, no. 1 (1977): 27–28.

Demello, Margot. *Animals and Society: An Introduction to Human-Animal Studies*. New York: Colombia University Press, 2008.

Dimeo, Paul. *A History of Drug Use in Sport, 1876–1976: Beyond Good and Evil*. New York: Routledge, 2007.

Francione, Gary L. "Animals as Property." *Animal Law* 2 (1996): i–vi.

Francione, Gary L. *Animals, Property, and the Law*. Philadelphia: Temple University Press, 1995.

Frederick, Joanna M. "Saving Silent Sufferers: The Case for Federal Regulation of Drug Use in Horseracing." *Mississippi Sports Law Review* 1 (2011/2012): 411–434.

Friedman, Bradley S. "Oats, Water, Hay and Everything Else: The Regulation of Anabolic Steroids in Thoroughbred Horse Racing." *Animal Law* 16 (2009): 123–152.

Gilbert, Michelle, and James Gillett. "Equine Athletes and Interspecies Sport." *International Review for the Sociology of Sport* 47, no. 5 (2012): 632–643.

Gleaves, John. "Enhancing the Odds: Horse Racing, Gambling and the First Anti-doping Movement in Sport, 1889–1911." *Sport in History* 32, no. 1 (2012): 26–52.

Haight, Walter. 1961. "Horses and People – No Butazolidin [*sic*] in Preakness." *Washington Post*, June 18.

Hankin, Susan J. "Not a Living Room Sofa: Changing the Legal Status of Companion Animals." *Rutgers Journal of Law and Public Policy* 4 (2007): 314–410.

Hauser, Marc D., Fiery Cushman, and Matthew Kamen, eds. *People, Property, or Pets?* West Lafayette, IN: Purdue University Press, 2006.

Hedenborg, Susanna, and Manon Hedenborg White. "Changes and Variations in Patterns of Gender Relations in Equestrian Sports during the Second Half of the Twentieth Century." *Sport in Society* 15, no. 3 (2012): 302–319.

Higgins, A. J. "From Ancient Greece to Modern Athens: 3000 Years of Doping in Competition Horses." *Journal of Veterinary Pharmacology and Therapeutics* 29 (2006): 4–8.

Hoberman, John. *Mortal Engines: The Science of Performance and the Dehumanisation of Sport*. New York: Free Press, 1992.

Hoberman, John. *Testosterone Dreams: Rejuvenation, Aphrodisia, Doping*. Berkeley: University of California Press, 2005.

Howland, Joan S. "Let's Not Spit the Bit in Defense of the Law of the Horse: The Historical and Legal Development of American Thoroughbred Racing." *Marquette Sports Law Review* 14 (2004): 473–507.

Hribal, Jason C. "Animals, Agency, and Class: Writing the History of Animals from Below." *Human Ecology Review* 14, no. 1 (2007): 101–112.

Huggins, Mike. *Flat Racing and English Society, 1790–1914: A Social and Economic History*. London: Frank Cass, 2000.

Huggins, Mike. *Horseracing and the British, 1919–1939*. Manchester, UK: Manchester University Press, 2004.

Huggins, Mike. "'Mingled Pleasure and Speculation': The Survival of the Enclosed Racecourses on Teesside, 1855–1902." *British Journal of Sports History* 3, no. 2 (1986): 158–172.

Huggins, Mike. "The Proto-Globalisation of Horseracing, 1730–1900: Anglo–American Interconnections." *Sport in History* 29, no. 3 (2009): 367–391.

Hunt, Thomas M. *Drug Games: The International Olympic Committee and the Politics of Doping, 1960–2008*. Austin: University of Texas Press, 2011.

Kay, Joyce. "Still Going After All These Years: Text, Truth and the Racing Calendar." *Sport in History* 29, no. 3 (2009): 353–366.

Kelch, Thomas G. "Toward a Non-property Status for Animals." *NYU Environmental Law Journal* 6 (1997): 531–585.
Kluesner, Amy L. (Williams). "And They're Off: Eliminating Drug Use in Thoroughbred Racing." *Harvard Journal of Sports and Entertainment Law* 3, no. 2 (2012): 297–321.
Labrie, Rose. *Dancer's Image: The Story of a Gallant Kentucky Derby Winner*. Woolwich, ME: TBW Books, 1982.
Landry, Donna. *Noble Brutes: How Eastern Horses Transformed English Culture*. Baltimore: John Hopkins University Press, 2008.
Leggett, William. 1960. "The Mysterious Buty Treatment." *Sports Illustrated*, August 1.
Liebman, Bennett. "The Trainer Responsibility Rule in Horse Racing." *Virginia Sports and Entertainment Law Journal* 7 (2007): 1–39.
Madden, Raymond. "Imagining the Greyhound: 'Racing' and 'Rescue' Narratives in a Human and Dog Relationship." *Continuum: Journal of Media and Cultural Studies* 24, no. 4 (2010): 503–515.
McEvoy, John. *Great Horse Racing Mysteries: True Tales from the Track*. Lexington, KY: Blood-Horse, 2000.
McFarl, Sarah E., Ryan Hediger, and Sarah E. McFarland, eds. *Animals and Agency: An Interdisciplinary Exploration*. Leiden, The Netherlands: Brill, 2009.
McManus, Phil, and Daniel Montoya. "Toward New Understandings of Human–Animal Relationships in Sport: A Study of Australian Jumps Racing." *Social and Cultural Geography* 13, no. 4 (2012): 399–420.
Milbert, Neil. 1971. "Boycott Off: Racing Today at Arlington; Heed Advice of Attorney to Follow Rules." *Chicago Tribune*, June 11.
Milbert, Neil. 1971. "Turf Storm Over Drug Evaporates." *Chicago Tribune*, May 12.
Möller, Verner. *The Ethics of Doping and Anti-doping: To Redeem the Soul of Sport*. New York: Routledge, 2009.
Möller, Verner. *The Scapegoat – About the Expulsion of Michael Rasmussen from the Tour de France 2007 and Beyond*. Odense: Peoples Press, 2011.
Nelson, Richard K. *Heart and Blood: Living with Deer in America*. New York: A.A. Knopf [Distributed by Random House], 1997.
Novak, Claire. "The Derby Drug Positive Protocol." *Kentucky Confidential*, May 11, 2011. http://kentuckyconfidential.com/2011/05/06/the-derby-drug-positive-protocol/
Nunalee, Mary Margaret McEachern, and G. Robert Weedon. "Modern Trends in Veterinary Malpractice: How Our Evolving Attitudes Toward Non-human Animals Will Change Veterinary Medicine." *Animal Law* 10 (2004): 125–160.
Plattner, Andy. "History of the National HBPA, Part III: Racing and the HBPA Step Into the Future." *Horsemen's Journal*, Fall 2003 http://www.hbpa.org/newsdisplay.asp?section=3&key1=1981
Ritvo, Harriet. *The Animal Estate: The English and Other Creatures in the Victorian Age*. Cambridge, MA: Harvard University Press, 1987.
Ritvo, Harriet. "History and Animal Studies." *Society and Animals* 10, no. 4 (2002): 403–406.
Rivera, Thomas. 1968. "Vet Hits Handling of Dancer's Image." *Chicago Tribune*, August 18.
Root, William C. "Man's Best Friend: Property or Family Member – An Examination of the Legal Classification of Companion Animals and Its Impact on Damages Recoverable for Their Wrongful Death or Injury." *Villanova Law Review* 47 (2002): 423–450.
Rothfels, Nigel, ed. *Representing Animals*. Bloomington: Indiana University Press, 2002.
Scott, Jason R. "Death to Poochy: A Comparison of Historical and Modern Frustrations Faced by Owners of Injured or Killed Pet Dogs." *University of Missouri – Kansas City Law Review* 75 (2006): 569–591.
Seinfeld, Jerry. *I'm Telling You for the Last Time*. New York: Universal Records, 1998. Compact disc.
Squires, Jim. *Headless Horsemen: A Tale of Chemical Colts, Subprime Sales Agents, and the Last Kentucky Derby on Steroids*. New York: Times Books, 2009.
Steward, Helen. "Animal Agency." *Inquiry* 52 (2009): 217–231.
Tobin, Thomas. *Drugs and the Performance Horse*. Springfield, IL: Charles C. Thomas, 1981.
Toby, Milton C. *Dancer's Image: The Forgotten Story of the 1968 Kentucky Derby*. Charleston, SC: History Press, 2011.
Todd, Terry. "Anabolic Steroids: The Gremlins of Sport." *Journal of Sport History* 14, no. 1 (1987): 87–107.

Tower, Whitney. "And the Last was First; Dancer's Image at Kentucky Derby." *Sports Illustrated*, May13 1968.
Tower, Whitney. 1968. "It Was a Bitter Pill." *Sports Illustrated*, May 20.
Tuan, Yi-fu. *Dominance and Affection: The Making of Pets*. New Haven, CT: Yale University Press, 1984.
Vamplew, Wray. "Sporting Innovation: The American Invasion of the English Turf and Links, 1895–1905." *Sport History Review* 35, no. 2 (2004): 122–136.
Vamplew, Wray. *The Turf: A Social and Economic History of Horse Racing*. London: Allen Lane, 1976.
Vamplew, Wray. "Unsporting Behavior: The Control of Football and Horseracing Crowds in England, 1875–1914." *Sports Violence* 1875–1914 (1983): 21–31.
Waddington, Ivan. *Sport, Health, and Drugs: A Critical Sociologocial Perspective*. London: Taylor & Francis, 2000.

Minor Problems: The Recognition of Young Athletes in the Development of International Anti-Doping Policies

Sarah Teetzel[a] and Marcus Mazzucco[b]

[a]*Faculty of Kinesiology and Recreation Management, University of Manitoba, Canada;*
[b]*Independent Researcher*

This article examines the role of young athletes in the development of the anti-doping movement in sport. In the law and ethics literature, children are considered a vulnerable population in need of special consideration and protection. Yet historically they have not always been treated as such, and in sport many rules apply universally to all competitors regardless of the participants' ages. This article provides a historical examination of drug testing policies created by the International Olympic Committee and World Anti-Doping Agency as they relate to minors as a means to uncover the ways in which anti-doping organisations have included age as a variable warranting special consideration. Challenges to anti-doping sanctions based on athletes' ages demonstrate that sport organisations, including the Court of Arbitration for Sport, have not placed much emphasis on the protected status of child athletes. This article situates children and youth in the history of drug testing policies and demonstrates how the unique rights of child athletes have been both managed and neglected.

Introduction

Examples abound of child athletes competing at the highest levels of competition, including the Olympic Games. Figure skater Sonja Henie was 11 at the time of her Olympic debut, and gymnast Nadia Comaneci was 14 when she achieved the first perfect 10 in Olympic gymnastics. Another 14-year-old, Aileen Riggen, won the women's diving event in 1920 in Antwerp, and diver Fu Mingxia was only 13 when she won the 10 metre platform diving event in 1992 at the Olympic Games in Barcelona.[1] According to most legal and philosophical definitions of 'children' and 'childhood', which will be discussed later in this paper, these Olympians were children at the time of their success.

Cases of young athletes caught using banned performance-enhancing drugs are not unheard of in sport.[2] Often the pressures to succeed start at an early age if an athlete shows signs of talent. The Youth Olympic Games (YOG) add to the pressure to set records and achieve victory that young athletes competing in regional, national and international events in age group, youth and junior categories face. The inaugural YOG, held in Singapore in 2010, were open to athletes aged 15–18 years on December 31, 2010.[3] All medallists as well as athletes selected at random were subjected to doping control. The testing netted two doping violations, both involving male wrestlers and the diuretic furosemide. Johnny Pilay of Ecuador and Nurbek Hakkulov of Uzbekistan, both 17 years old at the time, were disqualified from the YOG and required to return their participation certificates.[4] As Hakkulov's performance earned him the silver medal in the boys Greco–Roman 50 kg event, he was required to return the medal. A statement released by the International Olympic Committee (IOC) after the doping violations were announced called for an investigation into the role of the athletes' coaches, doctors and other support personnel, as well as the recognition that 'the two young athletes should be provided with some additional support and information on the danger of doping'.[5] Both athletes received two-year suspensions from sport.[6]

Pilay and Hakkulov were not the first young athletes to fail doping tests at major international competitions and, prior to their anti-doping violations at the YOG, two young athletes had committed violations at the Olympics.[7] The first was 16-year-old American swimmer Rick DeMont who lost his 400-metre freestyle gold medal at the 1972 Olympic Games in Munich after his urine sample tested positive for ephedrine.[8] Due to his asthmatic condition he required the drug Marax to breathe properly, which his team physicians failed to inform the Munich doping control officers until well after his doping violation was announced.[9] Despite appeals to the IOC Medical Commission by the US team physician Winston Rhiel and the US Olympic Committee president Cliff Buck, De Mont's punishment stood in spite of his age, his known asthmatic condition and the outrage expressed by members of the IOC and the public at his disqualification. Moreover, his doping violation led to ephedrine-containing asthma medications being permitted at the 1976 Olympics in Montréal.[10]

A second instance of a minor committing a doping rule violation at the Olympics involves Romanian artistic gymnast Andreea Răducan who was 16 years old when she competed at the Sydney 2000 Olympics. On September 21, Răducan took a Nurofen Cold and Flu tablet given to her by her team physician to ease her cold symptoms prior to competing in the Women's Individual All-Around Event. After winning gold she was sent to the doping control area to provide a urine sample. On September 24, Răducan competed in the final of the Women's Vault Event where she won the silver medal. She provided another urine sample after this event, which was found to be negative for all banned substances. However, both her 'A' and 'B' samples provided after she won the gold medal three days prior tested positive for pseudoephedrine, which was on the Olympic Movement's Anti-Doping Code's list of prohibited substances and an ingredient in the Nurofen tablets provided by her physician. The IOC disqualified Răducan from the Women's Individual All-Around Event, and ordered the National Olympic Committee of Romania to return the gold medal and the diploma awarded to Răducan for her first place finish.

Răducan filed an application to the Court of Arbitration for Sport (CAS) ad hoc division requesting the restoration of her gold medal, on the basis that she bore no responsibility for a violation since the Nurofen pills were provided by her team physician. In its decision, the CAS arbitrators noted that an anti-doping violation is a strict liability offence requiring no intentional element because the mere presence of a prohibited substance in a urine sample is sufficient.[11] Thus, the CAS arbitrators concluded that (1) an anti-doping violation had occurred and (2) Răducan's status as a minor did not alter the finding that she committed a doping offence because the Olympic Movement's Anti-Doping Code treats athletes of different ages alike.[12] Răducan was required to return her gold medal, but received no further disciplinary sanction. The CAS decision acknowledged that, in balancing the interests of the athlete with the commitment of the Olympic Movement to drug-free sport, the Anti-Doping Code must be enforced without compromise.[13] Acknowledging Răducan's unintentional doping violation, Jacques Rogge, who was a member of the IOC Executive Board at the time, noted:

> This is one of the worst experiences I have had in my Olympic life. Having to strip the gold medal from the individual gymnastic champion for something she did not intentionally do is very tough. But the rules are the rules.[14]

Rogge's comment encapsulates the formalistic adherence to the rules that is pervasive throughout the history of doping in sport.

The World Anti-Doping Agency (WADA), established in 1999, takes a strict stance when any athlete, regardless of his or her age, commits an anti-doping violation. This stance is demonstrated by the recent case of a 12-year-old Polish athlete Igor Walilko's positive test and subsequent ban from sport for consuming nikethamide, a substance found in some energy bars. After the Federation Internationale de L'Automobile banned Walilko for two years, a lawyer representing the child explained, 'He was very famous in Poland and, one day after, he was a criminal child'.[15] His lawyer argued, 'because Igor was under the age for the Youth Olympic Games cutoff, he cannot be considered criminally liable for doping'.[16] In June 2010, CAS overturned WADA's two-year suspension, noting it was 'excessive and disproportionate', yet the arbitrator hearing the case rejected the lawyer's claim that the athlete was too young to receive a doping sanction, and instead awarded a sanction of 18 months.[17] Applying an 18-month ban to a 12-year-old boy demonstrates that children are not immune to consequences for violating anti-doping rules. Unlike in many countries' legal systems, an athlete's status as a child often does not warrant different treatment compared to adults.

In the law and philosophy literature, children are considered a vulnerable population in need of special consideration and protection. Yet as the examples of DeMont, Răducan and Walilko's disqualifications demonstrate, many rules apply to all competitors regardless of their age. With the exception of restrictions that set upper and lower age limits for participating in specific disciplines and events, age rarely plays a role in high-performance sport. To help understand why anti-doping organisations have historically failed to consider age as a variable warranting special status and protection, past and current policies applied by the IOC, WADA and CAS are reviewed to examine the extent to which anti-doping organisations recognised age as a relevant factor in their decisions, and the implications of these decisions today. This article thus situates children and youth in the history of drug testing policies to demonstrate how the unique rights of child athletes have been both managed and neglected.

Minors, Children, and the History of Childhood

The idea that there is a clear distinction between children and adults has not been widely held across all cultures and times. Aristotle defined a child as 'an immature specimen'[18] that adults have a duty to care for and guide as he/she develops into an adult. Explaining the duty of parents and guardians to children, Shapiro contends,

> It is in virtue of children's undeveloped condition that we feel we have special obligations to them, obligations which are of a more paternalistic nature than are our obligations to other adults. These special obligations to children include duties to protect, nurture, discipline, and educate them. They are paternalistic in nature because we feel bound to fulfil them regardless of whether the children in question consent to be protected, nurtured, disciplined, and educated. Indeed, we think of children as people who have to be raised, whether they like it or not.[19]

Focusing on the distinction between individuals who are developed and individuals who are in the process of developing often serves as a demarking feature of the division between adulthood and childhood, but it is only a starting point.

From a developmental psychology perspective, adolescence marks the transition out of childhood that commences when a person reaches a state of biological, behavioural and social maturity, including 'the changed sense of personal identity that is occasioned by a transformed physique and altered social relationships, and the new beliefs about morality and the social order that accompany preparation for adulthood'.[20] Counter to theories of child development and socialisation associated with Piaget, Freud and others, Neil Postman argues convincingly that childhood is more realistically viewed as a social artefact rather than a biological necessity; that is, Postman suggests childhood was not discovered but invented.[21]

Based on his research on the history of childhood, Postman argues, 'the idea of childhood as a social structure did not exist in the Middle Ages, it arose in the sixteenth century'.[22] Postman demonstrates that conventional views of children as people in need of care and protection date back only four centuries to the Renaissance. Prior, in the medieval world,

> neither the young nor the old could read, and their business was in the here and now ... that is why there had been no need for the idea of childhood, for everyone shared the same information environment and therefore lived in the same social and intellectual world.[23]

Connected to the proliferation of literacy that transpired during the Renaissance, Postman argues:

> the [printing] press created a new symbolic world that required, in its turn, a new conception of adulthood. The new adulthood, by definition, excluded children. And as children were expelled from the adult world it became necessary to find another world for them to inhabit. That other world came to be known as childhood.[24]

Adulthood, by the sixteenth and seventeenth centuries, had to be obtained and earned through education, and was no longer simply something that happened as a result of growing older with the passing of time. The idea of childhood thus developed unevenly around the world: 'where literacy was valued highly and persistently, there were schools, and where there were schools, the concept of childhood developed rapidly'.[25] By the 1600s, common usage of the word 'child' included not only young people but also illiterate adults thought of as intellectually childish. Moreover, Postman explains:

> Almost all of the characteristics we associate with adulthood are those that are (or were) either generated or amplified by the requirements of a fully literate culture: the capacity for self-restraint, a tolerance for delayed gratification, a sophisticated ability to think conceptually and sequentially, a preoccupation with both historical continuity and the future, a high valuation of reason and hierarchical order.[26]

While a new concept of childhood had been established in the Renaissance, children unable to attend school continued to enter the work force at very early ages.

Social and cultural views of children in different eras shifted in response to changes in not only literacy and education, but also to changes in economic and working conditions, as well as family structures. In Western culture, the population shifts into urban centres that transpired as a result of the industrial revolution impacted family dynamics; for some young people, this resulted in protected childhoods, but for other young people, particularly in rural agricultural communities, their ability to labour made them vital members of the work force. The recognition of childhood as a time of innocence, separate from adulthood, was solidified by the end of the Victorian era as a result of attitudinal shifts that began to condemn child labour.[27] Often encompassed with efforts to improve women's social conditions and rights, twentieth century social reforms in many parts of the world have created interventions to protect children.[28] While specific age ranges demarcating children, youths, minors and adolescents vary from place to place, time to time and in different contexts, the United Nations (UN) uses a cut-off of 18 years to denote the beginning of adulthood. Article 1 of the UNs' *Convention on the Rights of the Child*, adopted in 1989, defines children as 'every human being below the age of eighteen years unless under the law applicable to the child, majority is attained earlier'.[29] Yet as the literature addressing the history of childhood demonstrates, this distinction is a simplistic and even arbitrary one. Today, sport policies do not routinely draw a line in the sand at age 18 to separate children and adults. For example, WADA defines a minor as 'a natural Person who has not reached the age of majority as established by the applicable laws of his or her country of residence'.[30] Many Sports Federations offer youth and junior events without a standard set of boundaries demarking the age categories or reference to legal maturity. In recognition of the history of childhood and the different ages at which humans are treated legally as adults around the world, in the remainder of this essay, we use the terms 'children', 'young athletes' and 'minors' synonymously to refer to all competitors who are not considered adults by their governments.

Children, Drug Use, and Doping

Reports of the use of performance-enhancing substances and techniques date back as far as records are available.[31] However, the ample body of literature addressing the history of performance-enhancing substance use in sport is largely silent about children's involvement, responsibilities and treatment. In the prominent sociocultural and historical anthologies and manuscripts addressing doping in sport (e.g. by Dimeo, Hoberman, Hunt, Møller, Schneider and Hong, Waddington and Smith, and Wilson and Derse), children are given very little attention or analysis, and none of these works contain a chapter, section or more than a paragraph dedicated specifically to young athletes' involvement with doping.[32] When children's involvement in the history of doping is included, it tends to be in conjunction with discussions of the anabolic steroid protocols forced upon some young athletes in the 1960s, 1970s and 1980s.

Translations of State Plan 14:25 Stasi files by Franke and Berendonk reveal that several hundred of East Germany's finest physicians and researchers administered unapproved experimental drugs to thousands of athletes, without gaining consent from the athlete or the parents of underage athletes. Their review of the classified military reports and publications for the Ministry of State Security reveals blatant disregard for the principles outlined in the Nuremberg Code and Declaration of Helsinki, particularly the importance of obtaining informed consent. They explain that 'several thousand athletes were treated with androgens every year, including minors of each sex. Special emphasis was placed on administering androgens to women and adolescent girls because this practice proved to be particularly effective for sports performance'.[33] Dimeo and Hunt demonstrate that 'doping was carried out in a way that was experimental, without the consent of the athletes or their parents, some of which included girls of childhood age'.[34] Yet these practices were not exclusive to East Germany, and teenage athletes from several countries are now known to have received banned substances.[35] Waddington and Smith draw on James Riordan's analysis of primary documents from the former Soviet Union to demonstrate that in several eastern European countries 'there had been long-term state production, testing, monitoring and administering of performance-enhancing drugs in regard to athletes as young as 7–8'.[36] These sources establish that adults provided a large number of minors with banned substances to fuel their performances.

Anabolic steroids are not the only substances banned in sport that have an association with use by children. The so-called braking drugs linked to female gymnasts attempting to slow down their bodies' physical maturity and the onset of the secondary sex characteristics associated with puberty are tied to minors as well.[37] Joan Ryan's analysis of elite women's figure skating and gymnastics provides insight into two sports subcultures that contribute to drug use by young athletes, not to enhance performance directly, but, through the use of laxatives and some banned diet pills and diuretics, to attain what the subculture considers the ideal and required physique.[38] In describing the extreme pressures these young athletes face to manipulate their bodies with drugs (and through starvation) to delay puberty in order to maintain girlish figures, an elite gymnastics coach interviewed by Ryan explains, 'gymnasts don't so much retire as expire'.[39] Thus, certain aesthetic-based sports, primarily for women, have an association with drug use by young athletes.[40]

The drug human growth hormone (hGH) also has a strong connection to children due to its intended use as a medical intervention to treat short children afflicted with malfunctioning pituitary glands. Three decades after scientists first extracted hGH from cadaver pituitary glands in 1956, scientists produced synthetic hGH successfully in the laboratory to meet the growing demand from parents of short children.[41] Demand for hGH grew in the 1980s due to strength and conditioning specialists' rumours of the drug's performance-enhancing benefits, as well as Durk Pearson and Sandy Shaw's advocacy of growth hormones as part of anti-ageing therapies.[42] The *Underground Steroid Handbook*, published and distributed by Dan Duchaine in the early 1980s, noted the effectiveness of hGH in stimulating muscular strength.[43] Duchaine's bold claims were analysed and contextualised in Terry Todd's article, 'The Use of Human Growth Hormone Poses a Grave Dilemma for Sport' (*Sports Illustrated*, October 15, 1984), which highlighted the risk to sport that undetectable hGH would entail. The IOC banned growth hormones and other peptide hormones in 1988, despite lacking a method of detecting these substances in urine samples.[44]

The American Academy of Pediatrics's policy on performance-enhancing drugs recognises that consumption of anabolic steroids, 'braking' drugs and hGH by healthy children poses a danger to young athletes. Established in 2005, the policy, which strongly opposes doping by young athletes, states that children constitute the most vulnerable population affected by doping.[45] A concern is that minors have not yet developed the advanced reasoning skills needed to weigh the potential benefits and harms involved in doping, and thus they cannot meet the standards for providing informed consent. The extreme financial and social perks that top athletes gain, as well as children's vulnerability to inducement and coercion, 'corrupt clear thinking in relation to the adolescents' future interests'.[46] Given the consensus in the legal and philosophical literature that children do not have the capacity to understand the magnitude of their actions, one might expect that the punishments and rules in effect when a child athlete commits a doping violation would be less severe and serve to educate rather than to punish. Yet an examination of the history of the anti-doping rules and policies demonstrates that this consideration was not at the forefront of discussions when anti-doping rules were being crafted and implemented.

WADA, the IOC, and the Absence of Children in Anti-Doping Policies

Prior to the creation of WADA in 1999, the IOC was the acknowledged leader of the anti-doping movement.[47] However, a review of the IOC Sessions and Executive Board meeting minutes, as well as the Medical Commission, Juridical Commission and Doping Committee folders at the Olympic Studies Archive in Lausanne related to the design or implementation of doping bans in Olympic sports, failed to uncover any discussion or recognition of children's status as a vulnerable population. Moreover, Hunt's thorough analysis of the IOC's involvement in anti-doping policy contains little reference to concerns or suggestions expressed by members of the IOC related to child athletes.[48] Thus, it appears that either children were not discussed at any of these meetings, or if they were, it was not in enough detail to warrant mention in the resulting meeting minutes.[49]

IOC members' discussion of children's rights and involvement related not to doping, but to the possibility of adding minimum age restrictions to specific events to ensure competitors were not young children.[50] From the first appearance of a rule regarding age in the French text of the 1924 *Olympic Charter* until 1977, the IOC stipulated that participation in the Olympic Games was not restricted to anyone based on age alone.[51] Yet at the 85th Session of the IOC in Rome in May 1982, the Athletes Commission's report included the recommendation that 'the introduction of a lower age limit is necessary in the interest of the athletes mainly for health reasons'.[52] The eventual decision to allow the International Federations to set lower age limits as each saw fit acknowledges a need to protect child athletes. Today the *Olympic Charter* clarifies: 'there may be no age limit for competitors in the Olympic Games other than as prescribed in the competition rules of an IF as approved by the IOC Executive Board'.[53] Very few other questions related to the appropriateness of subjecting child athletes to drug testing were found in the IOC meeting minutes. Instead, discussions frequently focused on unifying anti-doping rules, procedures and sanctions.

Current IOC publications do not address the issue of children doping in much detail either. In 2005, the IOC published its *Consensus Statement on Training the Child Athlete*, which declares, 'protecting the health of the athlete is the primary goal of the International Olympic Committee's Medical Commission'.[54] To this end, the consensus statement was designed to safeguard elite child athletes, which, according to the document, includes any young athlete 'who has superior athletic talent, undergoes specialised training, receives expert coaching and is exposed to early competition'.[55] These athletes are thus eligible for drug testing as part of WADA's registered testing pool. The consensus statement includes a review of the scientific literature on elite child sport participation and recommendations for ensuring 'the entire sports process for the elite child athlete should be pleasurable and fulfilling'.[56] In addition to discussion of burnout, overtraining and disordered eating, the document contains two references to doping. One is the statement, 'elite child athletes deserve to train and compete in a pleasurable environment, free from drug misuse and negative adult influences, including harassment and inappropriate pressure from parents, peers, health care providers, coaches, media, agents and significant other parties', and the other is that all athletes must 'comply with the World Anti-Doping Code'.[57] No further discussion of children and doping is included. The IOC's *Consensus Statement on Periodic Health Evaluation of Elite Athletes*, published in 2009, is similarly silent on concerns raised by child athletes' drug use, and health issues associated with child athletes are not specifically identified or addressed in this document.[58]

The first version of the *World Anti-Doping Code* (WADC), which came into effect in 2003, recognised the special status of childhood with the assertion: 'an anti-doping rule violation involving a Minor shall be considered a particularly serious violation'.[59] The 2009 update to the WADC includes the following additional information:

> while Minors are not given special treatment per se in determining the applicable sanction, certainly youth and lack of experience are relevant factors to be assessed in determining the Athlete's or other Person's fault under Article 10.5.2 [No Significant Fault or Negligence], as well as Articles 10.3.3 [Ineligibility for Other Anti-Doping Rule Violations], 10.4 [Elimination or Reduction of the Period of Ineligibility for Specified Substances under

> Specific Circumstances] and 10.5.1 [No Fault or Negligence]. Article 10.5.2 [No Significant Fault or Negligence] should not be applied in cases where Articles 10.3.3 or 10.4 apply, as those Articles already take into consideration the Athlete's or other Person's degree of fault for purposes of establishing the applicable period of Ineligibility.[60]

Article 10.3.2 of the 2009 edition of the WADC further specifies that athlete support personnel prescribing banned substances to minors will receive 'lifetime ineligibility' from further involvement in sport. The WADC and the International Standards published by WADA take a strong stand against adults who facilitate children's doping regiments, but otherwise do little to acknowledge a distinction between child and adult athletes.[61]

WADA's *International Standard for the Protection of Privacy and Personal Information* (2009) recognises that the drug-testing process requires athletes to disclose significant personal information. As a result, this document notes, 'Personal Information gathered in the anti-doping context can impinge upon and implicate the privacy rights and interests of persons involved in and associated with organized sport'.[62] The document specifies the rules and procedures that anti-doping organisations must follow to ensure they adhere to legal standards and maintain athletes' trust in their ability to protect their personal information. This document addresses children in one instance, noting:

> In cases where a Participant is incapable of furnishing their informed consent by virtue of their age, mental capacity or other legitimate reason recognized in law, the Participant's legal representative, guardian or other competent representative may furnish consent on the Participant's behalf for purposes of this International Standard, as well as exercise the Participant's rights arising under Article 11 below. Anti-Doping Organizations shall ensure that obtaining consents under such circumstances is permitted by applicable law.[63]

The acknowledgement that child athletes may not be able to consent to the collection, use and disclosure of their personal information recognises children's vulnerability and need of protection.

Children's vulnerability is also acknowledged indirectly in WADA's document, *Guidelines for Urine Sample Collection* (2010), which specifies that minors selected for drug testing are entitled to have a witness of their choice accompany them to the sample collection area and toilet to ensure the sample collection process is conducted appropriately.[64] To prepare young athletes for the possibility of being selected for doping control, the IOC now distributes a one-page handout for young athletes to familiarise them with the doping control procedures in effect prior to the YOG,[65] as well as a 37-page document for team officials.[66]

WADA's *Coordinating Investigations and Sharing Anti-Doping Information and Evidence* (2011) recognises the vulnerable status of child athletes with the statement, 'in cases of doping or non-sport use involving minors, and in order to reinforce their protection, there is a need for tougher sanctions for those who prescribe, supply, offer, administer or apply doping agents to them'.[67] A quote from the first president of WADA, Richard Pound, explains the rationale for imposing tougher sanctions on adults who enable children to break doping rules:

> The "upstream" organizers of doping on a broad scale, including traffickers and members of the athlete entourage, must be held accountable. They are well-organized and well-financed individuals and groups who prey on athletes and youth and who profit from cheating while risking very little themselves.[68]

Adults in positions of power in the sports world are forbidden from criticising the WADC or banned substance list in the presence of underage athletes. Mazanov, Connor and Hemphill caution sports medicine doctors that under a strict interpretation of the WADC, support personnel 'could face serious penalties for having a life saving, but prohibited, drug on your person or for expressing a critical view of the Code while in the presence of athletes under the age of eighteen'.[69]

The IOC and WADA's official publications are not the only doping policy guidelines that fail to differentiate concerns unique to child athletes. Many secondary sources that have drawn on the IOC and WADA's archival documents or provide critical analysis of these guiding policies lump all athletes together as one homogeneous group. For example, several reports prepared for WADA discuss children only in the context of preventive doping programmes that can be implemented to deter young athletes from committing doping violations.[70] The positions of sport governing bodies, including WADA, the IOC and some of the International Federations, regarding children and doping, can be interpreted further from the published decisions of athletes who challenged their doping accusations or periods of ineligibility by way of appeals to the CAS.

Sport Policy, Binding Verdicts and the CAS

The idea of the CAS stemmed from the IOC's realisation that domestic jurisdictions could challenge decisions made by the IOC and the International Federations. In an attempt to address his concern that 'instead of sport being decided on the field of play, it would regrettably spend more of its time in laboratories and courtrooms',[71] IOC president Juan Antonio Samaranch finalised the establishment of CAS in 1982, which the IOC as a whole voted to accept at its 85th Session in Rome.[72] Kéba Mbaye, a judge of the International Court of Justice in The Hague, led the drafting of the original statutes.[73] After the IOC voted to accept these statutes at its March 1983 meeting in New Delhi, CAS began operating in Lausanne, Switzerland, with the intention of 'facilitating the settlement of disputes of public nature arising out of the practice or development of sport, and, in a general sense, all activities pertaining to sport'.[74] The first case was heard in 1986.[75]

In functioning as 'an alternative to public judicial venues', Hunt argues CAS 'often undermined doping decisions by the IOC leadership'.[76] Instead of serving to protect doping decisions from reporters and the public, as was considered a perk of the CAS from the IOC's perspective upon its establishment,

> the body's decisions began to dilute the ability of the IOC to avoid unwanted interference on the issue. In a 1986 advisory opinion concerning the possibility of a lifetime ban for individuals caught using performance-enhancing substances, the CAS pronounced, for instance, that every action by an international sport body—including the IOC—must conform to basic principles of fairness; only *deliberate* offenses against legitimately promulgated and enforced rules and procedures would therefore warrant such a far-reaching punishment. While useful—and perhaps even necessary—for the protection of athletes' rights, such decrees provided significant obstacles to the type of tough countermeasures that many believed were needed by the IOC. In the longer run, though, these activities obliged Olympic policymakers to promulgate more rigorous standards for their own conduct.[77]

Now described as 'more than just an internal system of appeal that prevents sport from clogging up and getting clogged up in the ordinary court system',[78] CAS facilitates independent arbitration for sports-based disputes that arise from contractual and eligibility issues, and serves as 'the final checkpoint in the preventative process for doping in sport'.[79]

An examination of decisions rendered by CAS in past doping arbitration cases involving minors shows that the application of doping rules to child athletes is not based on the law of contract and its related principle of informed consent. Athletes are bound by doping rules by virtue of their participation in sport or their membership in a sport organisation. Thus, arbitrators do not view anti-doping rules as contractual in nature;

instead, they view them as 'quasi-legislative' in the sense that they apply to all athletes participating in a sport regardless of an athlete's ability to provide informed consent or legal capacity to enter into a contract. The only way an athlete can opt out of anti-doping rules is to stop participating in his or her sport. As a result, from a legal perspective, arguments that child athletes are not bound by doping rules because they are contractual in nature are unlikely to be accepted by CAS.[80]

Arguments that child athletes are too young to know or understand the implications of doping rules, or know what substances are prohibited, are often ineffective. In general, an athlete's age has no bearing on whether an anti-doping violation occurred. Moreover, an athlete's age also has no direct bearing on what sanction an athlete receives for an anti-doping violation.[81] The legal principle of proportionality requires WADA to create exceptions to the general rule that a period of ineligibility of two years is the sanction for an anti-doping violation. Two of these exceptions relate to whether an anti-doping violation occurred through no fault or negligence of the athlete, or no *significant* fault or negligence of the athlete. Yet the following examples suggest that in interpreting these exceptions, age is *not* a relevant factor that CAS arbitrators use *directly* in assessing fault.

CAS has dismissed anti-doping violations committed by young athletes in the past, but only under extremely extenuating circumstances. In 1998, CAS exercised its discretion not to impose sanctions or a period of ineligibility in arbitrating a case involving an asthmatic young handball player. The athlete (whose name and age are never specified in the decision, but who we can assume was under 18 due to the removal of his name from the public records) had taken Salbutamol to treat his asthma. In 1998, the Australian Handball Federation (AHF) had adopted an anti-doping policy that prohibited the use of most anti-asthmatic medications, except where it was taken by an inhaler only and when its use had been previously certified in writing by a respiratory or team physician to the relevant medical authority. One day after the anti-doping policy came into effect, the athlete was selected for a doping control test, and was unaware of the new rules. Prior to the test, the athlete informed Australia's Anti-Doping Agency that he had used his inhaler. Unsurprisingly, his drug test was positive for the prohibited substance Salbutamol. The athlete, the Australian Olympic Committee (AOC) and the AHF took the case directly to CAS,[82] where arbitrators held that the athlete had committed an anti-doping violation, but, based on extenuating circumstances, *including the athlete's age*, decided not to impose a sanction.[83] Most other young athletes appearing before CAS arbitrators to dispute doping infractions cannot match the level of extenuating circumstances demonstrated in this case, where it would have been unreasonable to punish the athlete. While this case serves as the only example we found where a young athlete received no punishment, it seems realistic to conclude that it was the unfortunate timing of the rule change, not the athlete's age, which led the CAS arbitrators to forgo imposing a sanction. Subsequent young athletes charged with anti-doping violations have not fared as well.

In the case of *S. v. FINA* in 2005, CAS concluded that an athlete bore no significant fault or negligence for using a cream containing a prohibited substance since she had received the product from her mother, yet imposed a one-year period of ineligibility. At the 2004 European open water swimming competition in Germany, a 17-year-old athlete tested positive for the anabolic steroid clostebol.[84] Her name does not appear in the CAS decision, but she is identified in the Fédération Internationale de Natation (FINA)'s *Doping Cases Report 1992–2005* (www.fina.org) as Italian swimmer Giorgia Squizzato. The FINA Doping Panel ruled that the swimmer had committed an anti-doping rule violation under FINA's Doping Control Rules and imposed a period of ineligibility for one year. Squizzato appealed to CAS, explaining she applied a cream, purchased by her mother, to her foot to treat a skin infection. CAS agreed with the FINA Doping Panel that the athlete had committed an anti-doping violation and that the period of ineligibility should remain at one year.

In the reasons for its decision, CAS noted that the standard two-year period of ineligibility in FINA's Doping Control Rules can be eliminated or reduced based on two exceptional circumstances: (1) if the athlete can prove that he or she bears 'no fault of negligence' for the violation or (2) if the athlete can provide that he or she bears 'no *significant* fault or negligence'.[85] In applying these two exceptions to the case, CAS concluded that although the swimmer was unaware that the cream she used contained a prohibited substance, she was nevertheless at some fault because FINA's Doping Control Rules state clearly that it is each athlete's duty to ensure that no prohibited substance enters his or her body.[86] The arbitrators noted that if the athlete had been more diligent, she could have realised that the cream contained a doping agent, since the steroid was listed on the cream's packaging and notice of use.[87] In addition, CAS also noted that the athlete's age (17 years) did not absolve her from responsibility because she had already been competing for 10 years at that time, and it is not uncommon to have 17-year-old athletes competing at the highest levels in swimming.[88] Citing previous case law, CAS added that 'age' does not fall within the category of exceptional circumstances for reducing a sanction.[89] Yet, CAS concluded the swimmer bore no *significant* fault or negligence, and therefore agreed to impose a sanction of one year. From this example, it is misleading to say that 'age' is not a relevant factor. Implicit in the arbitrators' reasoning was that the athlete was a minor. This is what made her reliance on her mother's advice reasonable.

One year later, CAS affirmed its position on doping violations committed by minors in its decision to uphold 17-year-old Belarusian artistic gymnast Nadzeya Vsotskaya's sanction. When the gymnast was selected for doping control at a world cup event in Belgium in 2006, her sample tested positive for the prohibited diuretic furosemide. She received a standard two-year sanction of ineligibility, but appealed to CAS to overturn the decision citing her age and reliance on her advisers. Her lawyer argued that, 'the Rules must be applied less rigorously and that a two-year suspension is a sanction too drastic and draconic, which may have the effect of ending Ms. Vyotskaya's career' because 'the average career of a female gymnasts is between 3 and 4 years. Thus, a two-year suspension has a much more significant effect on a gymnast that [sic] on athletes competing in other sports, such as equestrian or shooting'.[90] The arbitrators rejected the argument that the relatively short careers of elite women gymnasts should be considered in the awarding of sanctions, describing it as 'legally irrelevant'.[91] Furthermore, the arbitrators confirmed, an exception based on age 'is not spelled out in the Rules and would not only potentially cause unequal treatment of gymnasts, but could also put in peril the whole framework and logic of anti-doping rules not least in the light of the fact that in gymnastics (like in other sports) it is not uncommon to have minors compete at the highest level'.[92] Here again the reliance on a formal interpretation of the rules outlined in the WADC meant that the athlete's age, by itself, was insufficient to reduce or overturn her doping violation.

In a case brought before CAS by the Netherlands Doping Authority in 2009 to appeal the Dutch Appeals Committee's reduction of 23-year-old Dutch billiard player Nick Zuijkerbuijk's period of ineligibility to only one year after testing positive for the presence of Benzoylecgonine,[93] CAS restated its position on age. In its decision, CAS noted that it had already affirmed in previous arbitral awards that age is not a relevant factor when imposing a sanction, citing the following passage: 'it is not the age, sex, or any other personal characteristics of an individual that determines the application of the anti-doping rules but the participation of an athlete in the events governed by the rules'.[94] In doing so,

CAS clarified that the anti-doping rules do not distinguish between old and young athletes, and this statement has been cited in subsequent decisions.

One final example involves a case heard by the Sport Dispute Resolution Centre of Canada (SDRCC) involving 17-year-old weightlifter Chelse Zarboni-Berthiaume. When the athlete was asked to provide an out-of-competition doping sample at her training centre in 2010, she attempted to evade the test, and the doping control officers were unable to collect a sample.[95] She was thus charged with a doping violation. During the SDRCC hearing that followed, Zarboni-Berthiaume raised her age in order to justify her lack of responsibility in deciding to evade doping control. She claimed that she was a minor at the time of testing, and was subject to the parental control of her mother who did not allow her to provide a sample. She also claimed that, although she signed the 'Athlete Selection Order' form provided by doping control officials, she did not read or understand it or the consequences of refusing to provide a sample. The form specifies that refusing to provide a sample could constitute an anti-doping rule violation.[96]

In response to Zarboni-Berthiaume's argument, which emphasised her lack of informed consent and her age, the arbitrator applied article 10.5.2 of the WADC: 'While Minors are not given treatment per se in determining the applicable sanction, certainly youth and lack of experience are relevant factors to be assessed in determining the athlete's personal fault'.[97] The arbitrator concluded that the WADC 'allows an athlete's young age to be taken into consideration, but only to determine the existence or extent of fault, and not when considering the mitigation of the sanction'.[98] In Zarboni-Berthiaume's case, the arbitrator found that since she had admitted her fault by admitting she knew she was evading testing, her argument about being a minor did not need to be considered as the level of fault had already been determined.[99] Her claim that she did not understand the form she was signing, a key component of the informed consent process, was dismissed.

From these sport arbitration decisions, we can see that, in certain circumstances, an athlete's age is considered by doping authorities, but age alone is not enough to have a doping violation dismissed under the current rules.[100] These cases raise the question of whether enough weight is being given to age when determining the degree of an athlete's fault (and therefore, the length of a sanction), as well as whether age should be a separate exception under the WADC. It is not clear whether a blanket exception for minors would serve to recognise children's vulnerable status as open to influence and coercion by adults, or whether an exception of this nature would be inconsistent with the goals of the anti-doping movement.

Conclusion

While the ethical and legal issues associated with drug testing in sport have been well documented in the literature,[101] few of these concerns address the appropriateness of (1) holding child athletes responsible for their decisions to break anti-doping rules, (2) applying the same punishments to child athletes as adult athletes for committing doping violations and (3) subjecting child athletes to testing methods for which they are unable to provide informed consent. The rules governing participation in sports allow national and international anti-doping agencies to test athletes competing under their jurisdiction for the use of performance-enhancing substances because, no matter their age, all athletes are prohibited from using substances and methods included on WADA's Prohibited List. However, these rules do not seem to be in place to protect child athletes from harm.

Protecting child athletes is difficult when domestic and international standards addressing child rights are not recognised or adopted by governments. In many countries, 'sport organizations have historically been characterized as private bodies. They obtain their legal authority from their own constitutions, which are contractual in nature and confer upon them a self-regulating and autonomous status'.[102] The *Convention on the Rights of the Child* is one of nine international treaties adopted in 1989 by the UN, but it does not address sport directly.[103] International agreements, such as the *Convention on the Rights of the Child*, create a moral obligation for countries to respect. While the force of this document is moral, not legal, it can be used to 'provide the procedural means to inform policy development and best practices, guide the expansion of educational programmes and direct research initiatives'.[104]

Parental consent to analyse a child's blood or urine is sufficient in the context of health and medicine when the child's life or well-being is at stake, as per the Helsinki Declaration and subsequent medical research policies; however, sport is a voluntary, non-life-threatening pursuit. One might counter that parents or guardians willingly choose to authorise anti-doping officials to test their child's blood or urine because they feel doing so is worth the end result of possible athletic success. Yet adults' investment in children can lead parents, guardians and coaches not to act in the child's best interest. As Andy Miah points out, sport can become a coercive environment where the young athlete faces pressures that preclude him or her from making autonomous decisions.[105]

Child athletes sanctioned with a doping violation can face serious, lifelong ramifications. The damage that even a false positive test can have on a young athlete's career is highlighted by the struggles American swimmer Jessica Foschi faced in clearing her name after testing positive for the anabolic steroid meterolone in 1995 when she was 14 years old. Her sustained efforts resulted eventually in the doping charge against her being dropped, yet she faced years of suspicion as a result.[106] The stigma of a positive doping test can haunt a young athlete for the rest of his or her life. Part of many countries' doping deterrence strategies involves publicly announcing an athlete's name if he or she commits a doping violation.[107] However, in recent years, researchers have recognised the importance of values-based anti-doping education and messaging to reach young athletes, and instead of advocating for 'search and sanction' tactics that emphasise additional doping tests and punishments, call for better education as a form of deterrence.[108]

In other fields, such as medicine, education and research, children are considered a vulnerable population in need of special consideration and care, who are protected by guidelines and policies, including the Nuremberg Code and Declaration of Helsinki, which help ensure their protection from harms. Yet in sport they are not recognised with the same protection. The history of anti-doping policy development and challenges to anti-doping sanctions based on athletes' ages demonstrate that sport organisations have not placed much emphasis on the status of child athletes and their ability to provide informed consent. A strict liability approach to child athletes found to be doping is at odds with how children are treated in other spheres where they are recognised as a vulnerable population in need of care and special consideration.

The consent that all athletes give to anti-doping agencies to have their blood and urine analysed is not without some degree of coercion in the majority of cases, but particularly for child athletes.[109] While non-therapeutic research on children is heavily regulated and controlled by research ethics boards, drug testing young athletes is not covered by the same policies and protections.[110] If a young athlete breaches agreed-upon doping rules, additional implications arise in comparison to doping infractions committed by adults. Whether it is morally acceptable to subject youths to the tests used to detect doping in sport is unclear due to the ambiguity surrounding children and youths' level of autonomy, capacity to make decisions, and ability to understand the consequences and ramifications of their actions.[111] Children are unable to provide informed consent, but according to WADA, CAS and the IOC's rules, they can face the same repercussion and punishments for their actions as adults who have the legal competence and capacity to make informed decision. Recognition of child athletes' status as a vulnerable population given special status in most countries' legal systems seems absent in the world of sport. Additional analysis of how we ought to treat child athletes, specifically, is needed.

Acknowledgements

The authors would like to thank LeAnne Petherick and Russell Field for their assistance addressing the history of childhood. The authors would also like to thank the special edition editors and anonymous reviewers for their helpful comments.

Notes on Contributors

Sarah Teetzel is an Assistant Professor in the Faculty of Kinesiology and Recreation Management and a Research Affiliate of the Health, Leisure and Human Performance Research Institute at the University of Manitoba in Winnipeg, Canada. Her research interests focus on the history and philosophy of doping and gender issues in sport.

Marcus Mazzucco has a Bachelor of Physical and Health Education from the University of Toronto and a Juris Doctor from the University of Victoria. His research interests concern the protection of children's rights in sport, Canadian and international sport arbitration and international sport governance. Marcus is currently legal counsel for the Ontario Ministry of Health and Long-Term Care.

Notes

1. See Tymowski, "Rights and Wrongs," 58.
2. It is difficult to ascertain precisely the extent that child athletes have been associated with doping in sport. Privacy laws in many countries prevent the publication of children's names in public sources, and many decisions from the CAS remain classified and unavailable to the public. In this paper we discuss examples of child athletes associated with doping who received media coverage and/or are included in the public CAS repository. It is feasible that the number of doping violations attributed to minors is higher than we realise based on the available decisions. Researchers have been attempting to quantify the extent of the problem for several decades. Mike McNamee's analysis of the literature addressing youth drug use demonstrates that while it is difficult to pinpoint the percentage of minors who experiment with performance-enhancing drugs and substances, the prevalence of use is high enough to be of concern. See McNamee, "Beyond Consent," 111. Charles Yesalis's work, including an editorial in the New York Times in 1988, which identified steroid use by American adolescents for performance and aesthetic purposes as problematic, has been of particular influence in establishing youth drug use rates. See Todd and Todd, "Significant Events," 93; Yesalis, "Anabolic Steroid Use," 111; Yesalis and Bahrke, "Anabolic Steroid and Stimulant," and Yesalis and Bahrke, "Doping Among Adolescent Athletes."
3. Each International Federation participating at the YOG selects the age categories and events contested in its discipline. In 2010, 1678 young women and 1846 young men representing 204 National Olympic Committees participated in 201 events in 26 sports at the YOG. See IOC, *Fact Sheet,* 6.
4. See IOC, *IOC Disciplinary – Pilay*. See also IOC, *IOC Disciplinary – Hakkulov*.
5. "IOC catches 2 wrestlers doping at Youth Olympics" (*FoxNews.com*, October 15, 2010. http://www.foxnews.com/sports/2010/10/15/ioc-catches-wrestlers-doping-youth-olympics/).
6. Fédération Internationale des Luttes Associées. *List of Ineligible Wrestlers*. http://www.fila-wrestling.com/images/documents/anti-dopage/101209_list_of_sanctioned_wrestlers.pdf.
7. The web-based resources Sports-Reference.com and the Anti-Doping Database (www.dopinglist.com) were used to verify the dates of birth of all of the athletes committing doping

violations at the Olympics. We determined that only two athletes, Rick DeMont and Andreea Răducan, were under 18 years of age at the time of their positive tests at the Olympics. However, the number of doping violations committed at sports competitions outside of the Olympics is higher. Other doping violations will be discussed in subsequent sections.

8. Todd and Todd, "Significant Events," 71.
9. Hunt, *Drug Games*, 45.
10. Henne, *The Origins*, 22.
11. Arbitration CAS ad hoc Division (O.G. Sydney) 00/011 Andreea Raducan/IOC, award of September 28, 2009, para. 14.
12. Ibid., para. 22.
13. Ibid., para. 31.
14. "Court Supports IOC Over Raducan" (*BBC Sport Online*, September 28, 2000. http://news.bbc.co.uk/sport2/hi/olympics2000/gymnastics/944362.stm).
15. Martina Hyde. "The Smoking Athlete" (*The Guardian*, September 21, 2011. Accessed December 12, 2012. http://www.guardian.co.uk/sport/blog/2011/sep/21/doping-nicotine-drugs-wada-sport).
16. Emma Carmichael. "This Tween Polish Kart Driver Got Busted for Doping" (*Jalopnik*, March 30, 2011. http://jalopnik.com/5787326/this-tween-polish-kart-driver-got-busted-for-doping).
17. "Igor Walilko's doping ban reduced" (*ESPN.com*, September 15, 2011. http://espn.go.com/racing/story/_/id/6972514/teenage-kart-driver-igor-walilko-doping-ban-cut-cas).
18. Matthews, "The Philosophy of Childhood," para. 4.
19. Schapiro, "What Is a Child," 717.
20. Cole and Cole, *The Development of Children*, 619.
21. Postman, *The Disappearance of Childhood,* 143–4.
22. Ibid., 144.
23. Ibid., 36.
24. Ibid., 20.
25. Ibid., 39.
26. Ibid., 99.
27. For analysis of the connections between the disciplining of schoolboys and the creation of amateur sport, see Mangan, *The Games Ethics*. See also Sutherland, "To Create a Strong." The relevance of this connection to the history of childhood and sport was suggested by an anonymous reviewer.
28. Mayall, "The Sociology of Childhood," 243.
29. David, "Ensuring the Human Rights," 161.
30. WADA, *World-Anti Doping Code*, 130. Moreover, Petersen's examination of the athlete as role-model applies the term 'young people' to anyone under 21 years of age. See Petersen, "Good Athlete – Bad Athlete," 336.
31. For example, Veroken discusses the diet of dried figs used by Ancient Olympic competitors and the stimulants used by Ancient Egyptians and Roman gladiators in tracing the history of doping in sport back to antiquity. See Veroken, "Drug Use and Abuse," 1.
32. See Dimeo, *History of Drug Use*; Hoberman, *Mortal Engines*; Hoberman, *Testosterone Dreams*; Hunt, *Drug Games*; Møller, *The Ethics of Doping*; Schneider and Hong, *Doping in Sport*; Waddington and Smith, *An Introduction to Drugs* and Wilson and Derse, *Doping in Elite Sport.*
33. Franke and Berendonk, "Hormonal Doping and Androgenisation," 1262.
34. Dimeo and Hunt, "The Doping of Athletes," 588. Dimeo and Hunt provide the example of Birgit Boese, a former GDR athlete specialising in the shot put, whose state-sponsored doping regime commenced when she was only 12 years old, an age at which a child is clearly too young to provide consent. However, they argue that amongst the clandestine and coercive doping operations in effect in East Germany, 'there are also examples of athletes who knew what they were taking' (581).
35. Franke and Berendonk, "Hormonal Doping and Androgenisation," 1266.
36. Waddington and Smith, *An Introduction to Drugs*, 90.
37. In 1997 *Sports Illustrated* published an article mentioning 'brake drugs' that young women training to compete in gymnastics were alleged to be taking to stunt their growth and delay the onset of the secondary sex characteristics associated with puberty. See Michael Bamberger

and Don Yaeger. "Over the Edge" (*Sports Illustrated*, April 14, 1997. http://sportsillustrated.cnn.com/vault/article/magazine/MAG1009868/2/index.htm). The association of braking drugs with young gymnasts was raised by an anonymous reviewer.

38. Ryan, *Little Girls in Pretty Boxes*, 7. Ryan describes the pressures faced by girls training to be elite gymnasts and figure skaters to maintain 'missile' shaped bodies, which requires extreme effort on the part of the young athlete to delay puberty. She exposes the shocking number of gymnasts and figure skaters who died at young ages from injuries sustained attempting highly complex and dangerous moves to score high marks in competitions, and from the consequences of long-term anorexia nervosa and other eating disorders brought on by the pressures to be extremely thin and light in both sports. In discussing the real and perceived demands for female figure skaters and gymnasts to be as light as possible, Ryan shares the stories of several national, world and Olympic champions who abused diuretics, laxatives and diet pills, including pills included on the list of banned substances, to reduce their body mass.
39. Ibid., 34.
40. Many of the weight loss pills, liquids and laxatives female gymnasts can take to lose weight do not constitute or include banned substances or methods that lead to an anti-doping rule violation; however, the use of many products of this nature will trigger an anti-doping violation.
41. Prior to this time, growth hormones were available only in very limited supply because the only source was human cadavers. Holt, Mulligan and Sönksen, "The History of Doping."
42. Pearson and Shaw, *Life Extension*. This point was raised by an anonymous reviewer.
43. Duchaine, *Original Underground Steroid Handbook*.
44. Holt, Mulligan and Sönksen, "The History of Doping," 322.
45. American Academy of Pediatrics, "Policy Statement," 1103–6.
46. McNamee, "Beyond Consent," 115.
47. Ritchie, "The Spirit of Sport," 78–82.
48. See Hunt, *Drug Games,* 2011.
49. The historical records from all of the International Federations participating at the Olympics were not consulted. As one reviewer suggests, it is possible that more significant discussion of young athletes and doping might be found in the doping committee minutes of other sports federations, such as the IAAF or UCI; however, this possibility has not been confirmed.
50. Teetzel, "Minimum and Maximum Age," 340–7.
51. IOC, *Charte des Jeux Olympiques*, 13.
52. Minutes of the 85th Session of the IOC, Rome, 1982, Olympic Studies Centre Historical Archives, page 33.
53. IOC, *Olympic Charter*, 83. As a result the minimum age to participate in the Olympics varies based on the discipline. For example, athletes must be 14 years old to compete in taekwondo and bobsled but 17 years old to participate in wrestling, weightlifting and cycling events. See Teetzel, "Minimum and Maximum Ages," 343.
54. IOC, *Consensus Statement on Training*, 1.
55. Ibid.
56. Ibid., 3.
57. Ibid., 2–3.
58. IOC, "Consensus Statement on Periodic," 538.
59. WADA, *World Anti-Doping Code* 2003, 29. The same phrase is now included as Article 10.3.2 in the 2009 edition of the WADA Code.
60. Ibid., 58.
61. One other area in which the *World Anti-Doping Code* addresses youth athletes is with respect to education. Specifically the WADC states, 'To fight doping by promoting the spirit of sport, the Code requires each Anti-Doping Organization to develop and implement educational programs for Athletes, including youth, and Athlete Support Personnel'. However, a thorough analysis of anti-doping education campaigns is beyond the scope of this paper. See WADA, *World Anti-Doping Code* 2009, 14.
62. WADA, *Protection of Privacy*, 4.
63. Ibid., 10.
64. WADA. *Guidelines for Urine Sample,* 24. See also Canadian Centre for Ethics in Sport, "Annex 6C," 40.
65. IOC, *Doping Handout for YOG*.

66. IOC, *Anti-Doping Rules.*
67. WADA, *Coordinating Investigations*, A3-2.
68. Ibid., 7.
69. Mazanov, Connor and Hemphill, "2009 World Anti-Doping Code," 11.
70. See Backhouse et al., *International Literature Review.* See also Backhouse, McKenna and Patterson, *Prevention Through Education.* Moreover, Houlihan notes that early doping policy emphasised making lists of banned substances, identifying procedures for detecting these substances in athletes and establishing appropriate penalties for infractions. Yet in his thorough critique of doping policy development, he makes no mention of how organisations dealt with minors. See Houlihan, "Anti-Doping Policy in Sport," 318.
71. Anderson, "Sports Out of the Courts," 123.
72. Minutes of the 85th Session of the IOC, Rome, 1982, Olympic Studies Centre Historical Archives.
73. McLaren, "Court of Arbitration for Sport," 306.
74. CAS Statute, Article 1 as cited in Anderson, "Sports Out of the Courts," 124.
75. See note 73 above.
76. Hunt, *Drug Games,* 88.
77. Ibid., 89–90. Emphasis in original.
78. See note 71 above.
79. McLaren, "Court of Arbitration for Sport," 380.
80. In researching this paper, we did not find any CAS cases where this was argued, but it seems fair to assert that CAS will likely not accept this argument given its jurisprudence to date. Canada's dispute resolution body rejected this type of argument in the Zarboni case discussed later.
81. CAS arbitrations are typically decided on anti-doping rules, not international law. That is the point of arbitration. The parties have a dispute about a set of rules (in this case, anti-doping rules) and ask the panel of arbitrators to make sure those rules were applied correctly and in accordance with due process. Only in very rare cases has CAS applied broad principles of international law, such as proportionality, when interpreting and applying anti-doping rules. To date, CAS has not stated that the principles of informed consent or legal capacity to contract form part of international law that can be relied upon to decide doping appeals.
82. Australia's sporting bodies have rules that allow them to do this. Most other countries do not.
83. Arbitration CAS (Oceania Registry) A3, A4/00; AOC and AHF v. A., award of August 2, 1999.
84. See also Michael A. Hiltzek, "Athletes' Unbeatable Foe" (*Los Angeles Times*, December 10, 2006. http://articles.latimes.com/2006/dec/10/sports/sp-doping10).
85. Arbitration CAS 2005/A/830 S. v. FINA, award of July 15, 2005, para. 27.
86. Ibid., para. 33–7.
87. Ibid., para. 34
88. Ibid., para. 35.
89. Ibid.
90. Arbitration CAS/A/1413; World Anti-Doping Agency (WADA) v. Fédération Internationale de Gymnastique (FIG) and Ms Nadzeya Vsotskaya, award of June 20, 2007. http://www.wada-ama.org/rtecontent/document/CAS-2007-A-1413-Visotskaya.pdf.
91. CAS2007/A/1413 WADA v/ FIG & N. Vysotskaya, para. 83.
92. Ibid., para. 81.
93. A metabolite of cocaine that is on the Netherland's list of prohibited substances.
94. Arbitration CAS 2009/A/2012 Doping Authority Netherlands v. N., award of June 11, 2010.
95. Canadian Centre for Ethics in Sport. "Weightlifter Sanctioned for Doping Test Refusal" (*CCES Media Releases*, February 18, 2010. http://www.cces.ca/en/news-113-weightlifter-sanctioned-for-doping-test-refusal).
96. Due to varying testimony of different witnesses, the arbitrator decided that the athlete and her mother were not credible witnesses, and decided to accept the testimony of the doping control officials that the athlete attempted to evade testing.
97. WADA, *World Anti-Doping Code*, 58.
98. SDRCC DT 09-0114 (Doping Tribunal), CCES – and – Chelse Zarboni-Berthiaume – and – Government of Canada, WADA (Observers), para. 67.
99. Ibid., para. 70.

100. However, the CAS decisions that state age are not a relevant factor in assessing fault, or applying the exceptions to the general rule for sanctions pre-date the latest version of WADA's *World Anti-Doping Code*, which was released in 2009.
101. See Schneider and Butcher, "An Ethical Analysis of Drug Testing." See also Buti and Fridman, "Drug Testing in Sport," 1–5.
102. Mazzucco, "Using the Convention," 63.
103. See note 29 above.
104. Mazzucco, "Using the Convention," 68.
105. Miah, "Doping and the Child," 875.
106. Gregory Beaton, "Falsely Accused: Law Student Recalls Doping Charges" (*The Chronicle*, April 18, 2005. http://www.dukechronicle.com/articles/2005/04/19/falsely-accused).
107. For example, several national anti-doping agencies list all of the athletes currently serving doping-related suspensions from sport on their websites.
108. See Mazanov and Connor, "Rethinking the Management," 49. See also D'Angelo and Tamburrini, "Addict to Win," 700.
109. Munthe, "Ethical Aspects," 107–26.
110. Schneider and Butcher, "An Ethical Analysis," 144.
111. Teetzel, "Doping in Youth Sports," 41–60.

References

American Academy of Pediatrics. "Policy Statement: Use of Performance-Enhancing Substances." *Pediatrics* 115 (2005): 1103–1106.

Anderson, Jack. "Taking Sports Out of the Courts: Alternative Dispute Resolution and the International Court of Arbitration for Sport." *Journal of Legal Aspects of Sport* 10, no. 2 (2000): 123–128.

Backhouse, Susan, Jim McKenna, Simon Robinson, and Andrew Atkin. "International Literature Review: Attitudes, Behaviours, Knowledge and Education – Drugs in Sport: Past, Present and Future." Accessed January 9, 2013. http://www.wada-ama.org/Documents/Education_Awareness/SocialScienceResearch/Funded_Research_Projects/2006/Backhouse_et_al_Full_Report.pdf 2007

Backhouse, Susan, Jim McKenna, and Laurie Patterson. "Prevention Through Education: A Review of Current International Social Science Literature." Accessed January 9, 2013. http://www.wada-ama.org/Documents/Education_Awareness/SocialScienceResearch/Funded_Research_Projects/2008/backhouse_Prevention_through_Education_final_2009.pdf 2009

Buti, Antonio, and Saul Fridman. "Drug Testing in Sport: Legal Challenges and Issues." *University of Queensland Press Law Journal* 20 (1999): 1–5.

Canadian Centre for Ethics in Sport. "Annex 6C: Modifications for Athletes who are Minors." *Canadian Anti-Doping Program*. Ottawa: CCES, 2009.

Cole, Michael, and Sheila R. Cole. *The Development of Children*. New York: Freeman, 1996.

D'Angelo, Carlos D., and Claudio M. Tamburrini. "Addict to Win? A Different Approach to Doping." *Journal of Medical Ethics* 36, no. 11 (2010): 700–707.

David, Paulo. "Ensuring the Human Rights of Young Athletes." In *Sport, Children's Rights and Violence Prevention: A Sourcebook on Global Issues and Local Programmes*, edited by Celia Brackenridge, Tess Kay, and Daniel Rhind, 161–163. London: Brunel University, 2012.

Dimeo, Paul. *A History of Drug Use in Sport 1876–1976: Beyond Good and Evil*. New York: Routledge, 2007.

Dimeo, Paul, and Thomas M. Hunt. "The Doping of Athletes in the Former East Germany: A Critical Assessment of Comparisons with Nazi Medical Experiments." *International Review for the Sociology of Sport* 47, no. 5 (2012): 581–593.

Duchaine, Dan. *The Original Underground Steroid Handbook*. Published by the author, 1981.

Franke, Werner W., and Brigitte Berendonk. "Hormonal Doping and Androgenisation of Athletes: A Secret Program of the German Democratic Republic Government." *Clinical Chemistry* 43, no. 7 (1997): 1262–1279.

Henne, Kathryn. "The Origins of the International Olympic Committee Medical Commission and its Technocratic Regime: An Historiographic Investigation of Anti-Doping Regulation and Enforcement in International Sport." Accessed January 9, 2013. http://doc.rero.ch/record/17372/files/2009-The_Origins_of_the_International_Olympic_ Committee_Medical_Commission_-_HENNE_K.pdf

Hoberman, John. *Mortal Engines: The Science of Performance and the Dehumanization of Sport*. New York: Free Press, 1992.

Hoberman, John. *Testosterone Dreams: Rejuvenation, Aphrodisia, Doping*. Berkeley: University of California Press, 2005.

Holt, Richard I. G., Ioulietta Erotokritou-Mulligan, and Peter H. Sönksen. "The History of Doping and Growth Hormone Abuse in Sport." *Growth Hormone & IGF Research* 19 (2009): 320–326.

Houlihan, Barry. "Anti-Doping Policy in Sport: The Politics of International Policy Co-ordination." *Public Administration* 77, no. 2 (1999): 311–334.

Hunt, Thomas M. *Drug Games: The International Olympic Committee and the Politics of Doping, 1960–2008*. Austin: University of Texas Press, 2011.

IOC. *Anti-Doping Rules Applicable to the 1st Winter Youth Olympic Games in Innsbruck, 2012*. Lausanne: IOC, 2011.

IOC. *Charte des Jeux Olympiques*. Lausanne: IOC, 1924.

IOC. "Consensus Statement on Training the Child Athlete." Accessed January 18, 2013. http://www.olympic.org/Documents/Reports/EN/en_report_1016.pdf 2005

IOC, "Consensus Statement on Periodic Health Evaluation of Elite Athletes." *Journal of Athletic Training* 44, no. 5 (2009): 538–557.

IOC. *Doping Handout for YOG: Doping-Free Youth Winter Olympic Games*. Lausanne: IOC, 2011.

IOC. *Fact Sheet: Youth Olympic Games*. Lausanne: IOC, 2012. http://www.olympic.org/Documents/Reference_documents_Factsheets/The_Youth_Olympic_Games.pdf

IOC. "IOC Disciplinary Commission Decision Regarding Johnny Pilay Born on 17 May 1993, Athlete, Ecuador, Wrestling." October 2010. http://www.olympic.org/Global/Images/News/10-2010/15/SYOG001-Decision-DisciplinaryCommission.pdf

IOC. "IOC Disciplinary Commission Decision Regarding Nurbek Hakkulov Born on 13 March 1993, Athlete, Uzbekistan, Wrestling." October 2010. http://www.olympic.org/Global/Images/News/10-2010/15/SYOG002-Decision-DisciplinaryCommission.pdf

IOC. *Olympic Charter*. Lausanne: IOC, 2010.

Mangan, J. A. *The Games Ethic and Imperialism: Aspects of the Diffusion of an Ideal*. Harmondsworth: Viking, 1986.

Matthews, Gareth. "The Philosophy of Childhood." In *The Stanford Encyclopedia of Philosophy*, edited by Edward N. Zalta, 2010. Accessed January 15, 2013. http://plato.stanford.edu/archives/win2010/entries/childhood/

Mayall, Berry. "The Sociology of Childhood in Relation to Children's Rights." *The International Journal of Children's Rights* 8 (2000): 243–259.

Mazanov, Jason, and James Connor. "Rethinking the Management of Drugs in Sport." *International Journal of Sport Policy* 2, no. 1 (2010): 49–63.

Mazanov, Jason, James Connor, and Dennis Hemphill. "The 2009 World Anti-Doping Code and Medical Support Personnel." *Sport Health* 27, no. 1 (2009): 11–13.

Mazzucco, Marcus. "Using the Convention on the Rights of the Child to Protect Children." In *Sport, Children's Rights and Violence Prevention: A Sourcebook on Global Issues and Local Programmes*, edited by Celia Brackenridge, Tess Kay, and Daniel Rhind, 63–71. London: Brunel University, 2012.

McLaren, Richard H. "The Court of Arbitration for Sport: An Independent Arena for the World's Sports Disputes." *Valparaiso University Law Review* 35 (2001): 379–405.

McLaren, Richard H. "Twenty-Five Years of the Court of Arbitration for Sport: A Look in the Rear-View Mirror." *Marquette Sports Law Review* 20, no. 2 (2009): 305–333.

McNamee, Mike. "Beyond Consent? Paternalism and Pediatric Doping." *Journal of the Philosophy of Sport* 36, no. 2 (2009): 111–126.

Miah, Andy. "Doping and the Child: An Ethical Policy for the Vulnerable." *The Lancet* 366 (2005): 874–876.

Møller, Verner. *The Ethics of Doping and Anti-Doping: Redeeming the Soul of Sport?* Oxon: Routledge, 2010.

Munthe, Christian. "Ethical Aspects of Controlling Genetic Doping." In *Genetic Technology and sport: Ethical Questions*, edited by Claudio M. Tamburrini, and Torbjörn Tännsjö, 107–126. New York: Routledge, 2005.

Pearson, Durk, and Sandy Shaw. *Life Extension: A Practical Scientific Approach*. New York: Warner Books, 1982.

Petersen, Thomas Søbirk. "Good Athlete – Bad Athlete? On the 'Role-Model Argument' for Banning Performance-Enhancing Drugs." *Sport, Ethics and Philosophy* 4, no. 3 (2011): 332–340.

Postman, Neil. *The Disappearance of Childhood.* New York: Vintage Books, 1994.

Ritchie, Ian. "The 'Spirit of Sport': Understanding the Cultural Foundations of Olympism Through Anti-Doping Policies." In *Problems, Possibilities, Promising Practices: Critical Dialogues on the Olympic and Paralympic Games*, edited by Janice Forsyth, and Michael K. Heine, 78–82. London, ON: International Centre for Olympic Studies, 2012.

Ryan, Joan. *Little Girls in Pretty Boxes: The Making and Breaking of Elite Gymnasts and Figure Skaters.* New York: Doubleday, 1995.

Schapiro, Tamar. "What Is a Child?" *Ethics* 109, no. 4 (1999): 715–738.

Schneider, Angela J., and Robert B. Butcher. "An Ethical Analysis of Drug Testing." In *Doping in Elite Sport: The Politics of Drugs in the Olympic Movement*, edited by Wayne Wilson, and Edward Derse, 129–152. Champaign, IL: Human Kinetics, 2001.

Schneider, Angela J., and Fan Hong. *Doping in Sport: Global Ethical Issues.* Oxon: Routledge, 2007.

Sutherland, Neil. "'To Create a Strong and Healthy Race': School Children in the Public Health Movement, 1880–1914." In *Children in English-Canadian Society: Framing the Twentieth-Century Consensus*, edited by Neil Sutherland. Waterloo: Wilfrid Laurier University Press, 2000.

Teetzel, Sarah. "Doping in Youth Sports: An Examination of Privacy and Autonomy." In *Niñez, Deporte y Actividad Física: Reflexiones Filosóficas sobre una Relación Compleja*, edited by César R. Torres, 41–60. Buenos Aires: Miño y Dávila Editores, 2008.

Teetzel, Sarah. "Minimum and Maximum Age Limits for Competing at the Olympic Games." In *Rethinking Matters Olympic: Investigations into the Socio-Cultural Study of the Modern Olympic Movement*, edited by Robert K. Barney, Janice Forsyth, and Michael K. Heine, 340–347. London, ON: International Centre for Olympic Studies, 2010.

Todd, Jan, and Terry Todd. "Significant Events in the History of Drug Testing and the Olympic Movement: 1960–1999." In *Doping in Elite Sport: The Politics of Drugs in the Olympic Movement*, edited by Wayne Wilson, and Edward Derse, 65–128. Champaign, IL: Human Kinetics, 2001.

Tymowski, Gabriela. "Rights and Wrongs: Children's Participation in High-Performance Sports." In *Cross Cultural Perspectives in Child Advocacy*, edited by Ilene R. Berson, Michael J. Berson, and Barbara C. Cruz, 55–93. Charlotte, NC: Information Age Publishing, 2000.

Veroken, Michele. "Drug Use and Abuse in Sport." *Ballière's Clinical Endocrinology and Metabolism* 14, no. 1 (2000): 1–23.

Waddington, Ivan, and Andy Smith. *An Introduction to Drugs in Sport: Addicted to Winning?* New York: Routledge, 2009.

Wilson, Wayne, and Edward Derse, eds. *Doping in Elite Sport: The Politics of Drugs in the Olympic Movement.* Champaign, IL: Human Kinetics, 2001.

WADA. *Coordinating Investigations and Sharing Anti-Doping Information and Evidence.* Montréal: WADA, 2011.

WADA. *Guidelines for Urine Sample Collection.* Montreal: WADA, 2010.

WADA. *International Standard for the Protection of Privacy and Personal Information.* Montréal: WADA, 2009.

WADA. *World Anti-Doping Code.* Montréal: WADA, 2003.

WADA. *World Anti-Doping Code.* Montréal: WADA, 2009.

Yesalis, Charles E. "Anabolic Steroid Use: Indication of Habituation Among Adolescents." *Journal of Drug Education* 19 (1989): 111–113.

Yesalis, Charles E., and Michael S. Bahrke. "Anabolic Steroid and Stimulant Use in North American Sport between 1850 and 1980." *Sport in History* 25, no. 3 (2005): 434–451.

Yesalis, Charles E., and Michael S. Bahrke. "Doping Among Adolescent Athletes." *Baillière's Clinical Endocrinology and Metabolism* 14, no. 1 (2000): 25–35.

Who Guards the Guardians?

Verner Møller

Department of Public Health, Aarhus University, Aarhus, Denmark

The scope of this study is to document and discuss the vulnerability of athletes in doping cases – a consequence of the lack of transparency of anti-doping science, the strict liability principle and sport's arbitration system which denies athletes the possibility to have their cases tried in a proper court. After a brief presentation of the EU Athletes' call for involvement and change, this study introduces the concept 'corrupt idealism' which facilitates the understanding of anti-doping authorities' credibility problem. This study shows the historical prerequisites for the evolvement of this problem and presents and discusses a couple of controversial cases which expose the uncertain and pseudo-despotic nature of the system. This study concludes that an independent body financed by the working athletes unions should be established to oversee the work of anti-doping authorities and be involved in the development and administration of the anti-doping regulations.

Since the turn of the millennium, anti-doping has become a global industry. Many parties are involved and much money is at stake. The success of the campaign, in terms of public and political support, is based upon noble intentions: the protection of athletes' health and fair play. The dynamism between this idealistic goal and the occurrence of a number of high-profile doping scandals has leveraged an increasingly costly, intruding and vexing surveillance system as publicly criticised by some of the athletes subjected to it. Nevertheless, if we dare to rely on what most athletes say in public, athletes are generally supportive of the anti-doping endeavour.

However, in qualitative and quantitative studies, athletes have expressed concern over the efficacy of, and commitment to, anti-doping measures in other countries than their own.[1] This shows that athletes are not unanimously content with how the system works. Some athletes have started to question its fairness and reliability and, if actions are not taken to remedy this credibility problem, athletes may only grow more discontent with anti-doping efforts.

A stark reminder of this was the working athletes' meeting in Switzerland in November 2011, which gathered representatives from over 100 player unions representing more than 150,000 athletes.[2] The scope of the meeting was to form a global voice for professional athletes from all areas of sport. As part of this process, the World Anti-Doping Code was discussed and, despite being in favour of efficient anti-doping regulations, the EU Athletes' World Anti-Doping Agency (WADA) Code Review – a 102-page-long document containing the EU Athletes' written recommendations to improve the WADA Code – was astonishingly disapproving. The review expresses regret that athletes do not have a real say in the development of the regulations and explains that,

> The WADA Athletes Committee cannot represent working athletes on such a serious issue as anti-doping. With all due respect to the members of the Committee, it appears it is used more of a marketing tool as it is not independently structured, has no independent resources and has no collective mandate. The good intentions and stature of the participants does not overcome the fact that they may only express their opinions as individuals. If WADA portrays these individual opinions as the view of athletes in general it commits a serious breach of good governance and encroaches on the rights of player unions.[3]

Of even greater concern to WADA and everybody who sympathise with its course, the review continues by calling into question the legal foundation of the enterprise suggesting that,

> It is not consistent to fight for fairness in sport using means that contravene the basic "rules" of civilized society (human rights) [. . .] For working athletes, anti-doping rules and the resulting sanctions treat anti-doping rule violations as criminal in nature. Working athletes will lose their livelihood if they do not consent to anti-doping rules and therefore the consent is "non-voluntary". Likewise, the consequence for working athletes of imposed sanctions and public shaming can be a loss of their livelihood. A system that denies them their procedural rights (i.e. under Article 6 EHCR) may not be imposed. The current system is legally unstable and subject to challenge on human rights grounds.[4]

It is a regrettable fact that no penal system is perfect and never will be. Because humans are fallible, human judgement cannot be perfect. Every now and then judges make wrong decisions with devastating effect on the persons they judge. Therefore in civilised societies, ordinary legal systems have been harnessed by legal principles and procedures to reduce the room for mistakes and the risk of power abuse. Despite the separation of powers, the right to a fair hearing, the right to appeal and presumption of innocence, innocent people have still been put on death row only to be exonerated many years later due to new witness statements or new evidence.[5]

Because it is acknowledged that humans are imperfect judges and death is irreversible, the death penalty is regarded barbaric and thus abolished in all civilised countries except the USA. But the justice system as such is widely condoned as a necessary means to protect the order of society and individuals' rights. Mistakes are tolerated in the pursuit of the common good so long as they are understood to be unfortunate, unintended and exceptional. Rulers, law enforcers and judges are only legitimate so long as they exercise their powers unselfishly in accordance with the interest of the common good. This ought to be as true for sports authorities as for authorities in wider society.

However, the thesis of this study is that the world anti-doping system has historically evolved without proper recognition of the principles on which governing bodies legitimacy is based and, henceforth, today has become an unreliable institution with pseudo-despotic tendencies. This study is an attempt to show how this developed and to argue the need for an independent body – financed by the working athletes unions – to watch and control the work and decision-making of the anti-doping authorities and thus counterbalance the International Olympic Committee (IOC) financed independent body WADA.

The First WADA President's Response to Criticism

In his book *Inside the Olympics*, the former President of the WADA Dick Pound made a laudable observation: Officials, he wrote,

> must demonstrate that accountability starts at the top. Their own conduct in the management of sport must be, and like Caesar's wife, be seen to be, above reproach. They have a responsibility to act fairly, impartially and within the letter and spirit of the governing rules.

> [. . .] If the officials show no respect for the sport, how can the athletes and the public be expected to observe higher standards?[6]

Time and again, Pound has proven unable to live up to this ideal himself. During his presidency, he showed little patience with people who challenged the wisdom of the WADA-led anti-doping regime. His media spat with the world famous skier Bode Miller in 2005 is a typical example. One year after Pound had published the quote above, Miller presented his views on anti-doping calling the enforcement effort 'hypocritical, ineffective and invasive'.[7] During the same press conference, he argued that erythropoietin (EPO) should be legalised in skiing because 'in our sport, it would be pretty minimal health risks, and it would actually make it safer for the athletes, because you'd have less chance of making a mistake at the bottom and killing yourself'.[8]

Miller's viewpoint is indeed controversial but it is not unreasoned. As the winner of the World Cup and one of most successful American skiers of all times, Miller was a prominent subject to the anti-doping regime. So the least one could expect from Pound was (silent) acceptance of Miller's right to vent his frustration or a respectful counter-argument explaining why Miller's line of reasoning was mistaken if the President felt he was obliged to respond. Instead, Pound retaliated by an unworthy *ad hominem* argument: 'He enjoys his 15 minutes of fame . . . He's free to say what he wants. But it's irresponsible. It's just wrong', he fumed and fired a warning: 'If he says it during the Olympics we'll catch him and he'll perhaps have a different perspective than he has now'.[9] Pound's willingness to join the fray and make matters personal certainly cast doubt on his ability to live up to his own standards of impartiality and fairness.

To be sure, education of athletes is a commendable part of WADA's strategy. However, what Pound exercised with Miller is not education but mind policing, a prominent feature in totalitarian societies. It is understandable that Pound was annoyed that a high-profile athlete challenged the regime. And his outburst over Miller's opinions could be excused as a lamentable loss of temper had it been a one-off accident. The truth is, however, it had happened time and again. After a complaint filed by seven-time Tour de France winner Lance Armstrong, Pound finally received a reprimand from the IOC's Ethics Commission advising the IOC Executive Committee to remind him of his obligation as a member of the IOC 'to exercise greater prudence consistent with Olympic spirit when making public pronouncements that may affect the reputation of others'.[10] Not that this made Pound yield. Interviewed at the end of his WADA-reign he admitted that, 'his willingness to lob verbal grenades in the direction of certain athletes at the slightest invitation by the media' was part of his strategy and that 'he has no regrets about the enemies he has made along the way'.[11]

Since he stepped down, Pound has continued his fight for doping-free sport using his platform as a member of the IOC's Board of Directors to cast suspicion on well-performing athletes. In an interview with *Reuters* at the closing day of the London 2012 Olympics, for instance, he insinuated that Jamaica's world-class sprinters were doping. These comments came in response to the question whether he was satisfied with the way Jamaica tested its athletes. Pound admitted he was not because Jamaican athletes were 'one of the groups that are hard to test, it is (hard) to get in and find them and so forth'. He said so despite the Jamaican Anti-Doping Agency had 'never had a complaint from WADA that the agency was having problems locating any Jamaican athlete for testing'.[12]

In hindsight, it is tempting to maintain that Pound's offensive approach towards Lance Armstrong, Floyd Landis and others has been justified by the evidence and confessions recorded afterwards. Pound's insinuation that the outstanding achievements of the Jamaican sprinters is built on doping could be right as well. However, as likely as his reasoning may be, he does not have legitimate backing for his words. Thus, stating such suspicions publicly is against the fundamental principle presented by Pound himself in the quote above that officials 'must be above reproach' and 'have a responsibility to act fairly, impartially and within the letter and spirit of the governing rules'.

Even if Pound were the odd man out, the situation would still be disquieting given his status. However, there are indications that he is not alone. Anti-doping attracts people who are so passionate about the course that they are willing to bend the rules for the greater good and this makes the situation even more worrying. A prominent, albeit not exceptional example, as will be apparent in what follows, is the International Cycling Federation's former Head of Anti-Doping Anne Gripper who in 2008 accepted to reconsider the Russian cyclist Vladimir Gusev's urine sample in accordance with the new WADA standards after he had won his case against his team, Astana, for being unjustly fired in the wake of a suspicious test provided for the teams' internal anti-doping programme.[13] Gripper's willingness to help Astana, which the CAS ruled should pay Gusev €650,000 in compensation, indicates that the anti-doping course was more important to her than the letter of the anti-doping regulations. The previous year she had handled the Michael Rasmussen case with similar disregard of the regulations. When she realised that Rasmussen was exploiting the whereabouts system, Gripper handed him a warning stating that he had posted his update information 4 days late and decided to record the warning even though he responded to her written warning that he posted his update on time and she was in possession of the envelope which had a stamp on it that proved him right.[14]

It does not bode well for the protection of athletes' rights that – at least a significant fraction of – those engaged in anti-doping apparently see themselves as shepherds and think in accordance with the Enlightenment philosopher Jean-Jacques Rousseau's description that: 'As a shepherd is of nature superior to that of his flock, the shepherds of men, i.e. their rulers, are of a nature superior to that of the peoples under them'.[15] Rousseau found this view of management unsustainable and argued convincingly against it in his book *The Social Contract* originally published in 1762. Rousseau explains that voluntary and willed consent is the foundation for people's obligation to obey legislation. 'Laws are properly speaking, only the conditions of civil association', Rousseau explained, 'The people being subject to the laws, ought to be their author: the conditions of the society ought to be regulated solely by those who come together to form it'.[16] Accordingly, those who are entrusted with the executive power of the common will should be considerate and humble in the exertion of power and not take advantage of it to promote personal views, interests or agendas. WADA's persistent presentation of anti-doping as an effort to protect clean athletes right to compete in drug-free sport leaves the impression that the official anti-doping authorities agree with Rousseau's idea in principle even if they do not live up to them in practice.

The Corrupting Power of Idealism

Corruption is commonly associated with dictators who put away vast sums of money in secret bank accounts and powerful officials who use their position to favour friends, family or themselves. But there is a different breed, I will argue, that tends to go unnoticed, namely the 'corrupt idealists'. The corrupt idealists do not do any of the things that immediately qualify as corruption in the common understanding of the word. They are by and large decent, unselfish and well-respected people whose corruption occurs incidentally in the pursuit of what they in accordance with their own value system perceive as good for other people or society in general. When corrupt idealists identify a problem, whether it be a threat to the environment, to social cohesion, to the moral order, or unjust, abuse, discrimination or harassment of this or that group, they want to do something about it and their idealistic nature makes them loose sight of proportion. They become obsessed with the problem and determined to press on with what they think needs to be done to solve it as if they sensed a holy calling. The main characteristic of the corrupt idealists is that they are imperceptive of their immoral acts because they understand these acts as justified by the noble course. The mythological example of a corrupt idealist is Abraham who on God's demand instantaneously proved willing to sacrifice his only son Isaac.

Corrupt idealists may hold leading positions but can be found at all levels of governmental and non-governmental organisations. There are also corrupt idealists who work independently trying to influence organisations and policy-makers from outside. Pound's own admittance of his willingness to lob verbal grenades in the direction of otherwise untainted athletes, as part of his strategy to combat doping, is a clear-cut example of corrupt idealism. The distinguished Austrian sports physician Ludwig Prokop, who played a pioneering role in anti-doping during the 1950s, is another example of the same.

As a member of the IOC's Medical Committee Prokop became increasingly concerned about drug use in sport in the 1950s following various experiences. During the 1952 Olympics, he found syringes and broken vials in the speed skaters' locker room, and in 1954 he witnessed a strychnine cramp at the World Championships in weightlifting.[17] He was also aware of the drug-related near-fatal collapses that had happened in cycling. As sports historian Paul Dimeo demonstrates Prokop's main concern was not the athletes' health but the corruption of the ideal of fair competition. Regardless whether athletes' use of drugs was unhealthy or not, it was still unfair, he maintained.[18] Prokop approached the doping problem with such a view in mind. If athletes' health were the primary concern, he contended, the logical thing to do would be to promote the education of athletes to use the right medicine to retain their health under the extreme physical demands of sport. However, Prokop's 'pure sport' ideal required zero tolerance of doping, the end result he desired. As a physician, he was aware that moderate performance-enhancing drug use did not necessarily imply huge health risks, but he understood that the health argument would be useful to promote the course of doping-free sport.[19]

Hence, when the Danish cyclist Knud Enemark Jensen collapsed during the 100-km team time trial at the 1960 Rome Olympics, Prokop took Jensen's death as an opportunity to raise awareness about drug problems and advance his 'pure sport' anti-doping campaign that was still in its infancy. Without evidence, Prokop published a report claiming that Jensen died as a result of an overdose of amphetamines.[20]

Prokop's conclusion, however persuasive, was inaccurate. The official medico-legal report, based on the Italian forensics' autopsy and submitted to the Danish Police Authorities in 1961, revealed no traces of amphetamines and concluded that Jensen died from heatstroke. Nevertheless, because of Prokop's status and academic credentials many people trusted him. His version of Jensen's death took hold in the public imagination and lasted well into the twentieth century. Indeed, Prokop's personal assumption that amphetamines caused Jensen's death has been circulated so often in scholarly books and articles that it has gained status of historical fact. In an interview as late as 2001, the ageing Prokop admitted he had 'never seen documentation to prove that his death was caused by doping. Perhaps it was wrong of me to draw it out in the report', he reflects before he justifies his decision by emphasising that Jensen did not die in vain. 'Remember that Knud Enemark's death initiated the fight against doping.'[21] It is obvious that Prokop's anti-doping idealism allows him to compromise truth for the benefit of the greater good.

Prokop is not the only scientist who has valued rumours over evidence. Randy E. Eichner, a haematologist at the University of Oklahoma Health Sciences Center, has also turned myth into 'fact' for the sake of anti-doping. This time, it was the sudden death from heart failure, allegedly caused by EPO abuse, which struck a number of Dutch and Belgian cyclists in the late 1980s and early 1990s. However, media and communication researcher Bernat López trawled the literature in a meticulous study of the case and found that the myth originated from a spokesperson from the Dutch Cycling Federation, and a Belgian physician quoted in newspapers. But López did not find any reliable evidence to substantiate these sources' claims. López labels EPO 'the drug of mass destruction' because the loaded narrative that EPO was responsible for a number of healthy young athletes premature death echoes US President George W. Bush's unfounded 'weapons of mass destruction' justification for his invasion of Iraq. Lopez indicates that similar scare tactics to the war in Iraq helped magnify the doping problem and convince politicians that firm action was needed.

Eichner was one of the first within the scientific community to take advantage of this journalistic myth. His idealism is unmistakable in his writing: 'I am not so much concerned with getting the athlete to the finish-line first, but with getting him there alive', he said in 1990 shortly after the EPO myth had begun to disseminate.[22] Such comments not only made him out to be a sane voice amidst the insane world of sport but also allowed him to take the moral high ground. Yet Lopez quotes him as saying:

> The wife of Johannes Draaijer, who had died in his sleep in January 1990, stated that "her husband was against doping, that he was well known in the peloton as a non-user", and that "the [post-mortem] investigations showed nothing" that could relate Draaijer's death with EPO. But Eichner seemed to know better, as he showed no hesitation in dismissing Lisa Draaijer's opinions as "just a cover-up ... just something they've brainwashed her with".[23]

Regardless of Johannes Draajer's reputation and the content of the post-mortem, Eichner does not hesitate to dismiss the widow's defence of her husband's name. The persuasive effect of the 'drug of mass destruction' was apparently too good to leave room for doubt. Eichner was not the only scientist who took this position and debunked the post-mortem. Lopez explains that,

> Norman Gledhill, an exercise physiologist at York University in Toronto, made an equally bold claim targeting the forensics: 'There's either been a massive cover-up or the people who did [the investigations] were massively incompetent. I think the cover-up is the likely answer'.[24]

López names other physicians who willingly backed the EPO-deaths myth and sowed doubt about alternative explanations.

It is a well-known phenomenon in the history of science that scientists have lambasted theories that went against their own research, convictions or religious beliefs as Adam Sedgwick attack on Charles Darwin's theory of evolution and Arthur Patscke's refusal of Albert Einstein theory of relativity testify to. However, protecting a theory or a belief by criticising colleagues who present alternative theories does not qualify as corruption in any way. Simple corruption is coupled with intentional dishonesty. A key feature of the corrupt idealists, on the other hand, is that they do not understand that what they are doing is dishonourable. They usually see criticism as ill-intended opposition and are apparently immune to factual arguments that contradict their perception of the matter. López's investigation of Eichner's promotion of the EPO-myth exemplifies this:

> ... if one goes down the chain of quotations started by Eichner himself in his 2007 article, one finds not only a lack of empirical evidence for his claims about the fatal effects of EPO, but even an article based on original research that refutes Eichner's contention about the causal link between EPO and blood clotting, at least as far as vascular access is concerned.[25]

Unsurprisingly, anti-doping work attracts people who sympathise with the course. History has shown that corrupt idealists have dotted the anti-doping landscape. From scientists such as the above-mentioned Prokop and Eichner to adminstrators such as Brundage and Pound, zealots in hot pursuit of dope-free sport have exempted themselves from their own standards, always justifying their means by the larger ends they serve. Consequently, there is reason to believe that there are also corrupt idealists working with the development of the anti-doping testing and regulation. In the light of this, it is critical that anti-doping work is transparent in all facets of the management and development process.

Presumptuous Reactions to Scientific and Legal Criticism

Given the serious consequences it has for athletes to be found guilty of doping, one would hope that the control is based on the highest possible scientific standard. Because of the strict liability rule, athletes have no defence against a positive test other than by pointing to errors in the test procedure that can have caused the positive result. Therefore, it ought to be taken seriously when qualified experts voice concern about the quality and reliability of anti-doping science.

A review study by Guiseppe Banfi et al. found that anti-doping laboratory analytical methods are not properly standardised, which leads to incongruent data and thus increased risk of false-positive results. The authors suggest that anti-doping is not as safe and reliable as it should be and that WADA should take advantage of the valuable experience laboratory medicine has built over many years in pursuing quality and safety in the testing process. In line with this, they conclude that 'laboratory medicine must be involved in evaluating, validating and choosing methodologies, instrumentation and parameters'.[26]

Two years ago, the statistician Donald Berry raised similar concerns in a *Nature* commentary. Barry critiqued the insufficient application of statistics and argued that, for the test to be reliable, a large number of samples – both positive and negative – 'tested by blinded technicians who use the same procedures under the same conditions present in actual sporting event' should be known. But 'such studies have not been adequately done, leaving the criterion for calling a test positive unvalidated'.[27] Berry furthermore observed that the 'method used to establish the criterion for discriminating one group from another has not been published and tests have not been performed to establish sensitivity and specificity.' Thus, he concludes that 'if conventional doping testing were to be submitted to a regulatory agency such as the US Food and Drug Administration to qualify as a diagnostic test for a disease, it would be rejected'.[28]

Bearing in mind the devastating consequences it has for athletes to fail a test, Berry's far-reaching critique calls for careful response. *Nature*'s editor-in-chief understood this and proclaimed in his editorial that 'by not opening to broader scientific scrutiny the methods by which testing labs engage in study, it is Nature's view that the anti-doping authorities have fostered a sporting culture of suspicion, secrecy and fear' before he advocated that 'drug testing should not be exempt from the scientific principles and standards that apply to other biomedical sciences'.[29]

Interestingly, in the journal's next volume, there were three responding letters. Two of those – submitted by researchers with no stock in anti-doping – recognised the methodological problems identified by Berry and praised his commentary, whereas the third letter, authored by Pierre-Edouard Sottas and two of his colleagues at the Swiss Laboratory for Doping Analyses, was opposed to Berry's line of reasoning. Sottas et al. explained that anti-doping is not a medical but a forensic science and, therefore, not solely based on statistics. Moreover, a paradigm shift has taken place in forensics from 'the traditional assumptions of "absolute certainty" and "discernible uniqueness" in favour of an empirical and probabilistic approach'.[30] This shift has also influenced anti-doping as the introduction of the biological passport exemplifies. So rather than being 'on the wrong path' as Berry maintains anti-doping is actually on par with cutting edge research, the Swiss anti-doping analysts asserted before they rebuked the editor-in-chief with a remarkable accusation for his support of Berry's principled advocacy for good scientific practice: 'The role of anti-doping science is to protect clean athletes. Your Editorial may have just the opposite effect'.[31]

It is obvious that if Berry and other critics of anti-doping science are ignorant about how the regime really works, as Sottas et al. indicate, the critics should be corrected and informed. The most honest reaction to the critics would be to engage openly with the scientific community in the pursuit of the most efficient and reliable testing programme. Presumptuous repudiation and vilification of critics are detrimental to the credibility of the anti-doping enterprise. This, nevertheless, appears to be the anti-doping establishment's preferred strategy.

When in 2008 Carsten Lundby et al. published a study of the efficacy of WADA-accredited laboratories urine test for recombinant human EPO and found that it was not reliable, they too were discredited where they ought to be thanked by those who have the protection of clean athletes at heart. Such praise was due because not only did this study find false negatives, but it also found one false positive, an erroneous indication that a non-doped sample contained evidence of doping.

Lundby et al.'s design was as simple as it was bold. Eight male students were studied for 7 weeks. In the first 2 weeks (boosting period), they were given injections with 5000 units of EPO every other day. In the following, 2 weeks (maintenance period), they were given the same dose once a week. In the last 3 weeks of the study (post period), the subjects were not given any EPO but were still providing urine samples. All urine samples were divided into two and sent to two different WADA-accredited laboratories following the standard procedure for storing and transportation of the samples. Laboratory A detected EPO in all the samples in the boosting period whereas laboratory B found no positives. Laboratory B reported one sample 'negative' while seven were reported 'suspicious', which according to WADA's protocol would not result in a doping case. The detection during the maintenance and post period, where haemoglobin mass and performance level were elevated, was really poor. Laboratory B found no positive or suspicious at all and laboratory A only found 2 of 24 to be positive and 3 to be suspicious. However, the most controversial finding was that one test person was reported negative on day 30 (2 days after his last EPO injection) but positive on day 35 (7 days after his last EPO injection), which appeared to confirm 'cases of false-positive testing in an experimental setting'.[32]

The reaction to this study was similar to the reaction to Berry's commentary. Members of the scientific community with no stock in anti-doping wrote letters to the editor which approved the study and provided additional information to support the claim that the urine test for EPO was 'tilting at windmills' (Jelkmann 2008). Those who were responsible for the laboratory tests, on the other hand, came out defending their territory accusing the authors of scientific malpractice. Martial Saugy et al. responsible for the alleged false-positive test at the WADA-accredited laboratory in Switzerland went so far as to conclude that,

> the published results cannot be credited with any scientific credibility and demonstrate a great lack of knowledge of the authors regarding the EPO detection method and, more generally, of the whole anti-doping procedures. This publication has to be considered as a major offense to

the scientists working years to help the sports authorities to efficiently deal with doping in their disciplines.[33]

It is unsurprising that the laboratory scientists responsible for the test felt exposed and did their best to explain away the disastrous results. But if the scientists behind the controversial experiment lacked knowledge about the EPO detection, the reason must be that there are things about the test analysis method that are kept secret even to the laboratory's external partners since Saugy et al. admit that: 'Since spring 2006, the laboratory of Lausanne [Laboratory A] has been collaborating with the group of Lundby et al.'.[34] Hence, improved transparency of anti-doping and open engagement with the scientific community about evaluating, validating and choosing (new) methodologies, as Banfi called for above, appear to be the ethical way to remedy the WADA-accredited laboratories credibility crises.

The obvious argument against improved transparency is that if every aspect of the test and the analysis procedure was published, it would make it easier for those who assist athletes doping to beat the system. But this is a pragmatic argument that devalues good scientific practice. Lundby et al.'s 'partisan' study shed light on the dilemma. Either you publish everything and accept that independent scientists can test the quality of the tests and help improve testing, which poses risks that those who work on the 'dark side' in practice falsify the test and without publication invent methods by which they can beat the system. Or you accept that athletes are subject to a suboptimal anti-doping control system developed in the dark, which produces a high number of false negatives and an unknown number of false positives.

After the publication of his study, Lundby was informed by a senior person in WADA's scientific committee that he should not bother applying for WADA funding in the future because if he did, it would be a waste of time for both himself and WADA. In an interview with *Weekendavisen*, a Danish equivalent to *Newsweek*, Lundby further explained the consequence of the malign relationship between WADA 'in-house' researchers and the independent research community:

> Most of my international colleagues are tired of WADA. We consider it to be a bunch of friends who go around and pat each other on their backs. I do not want to deal with anti-doping work anymore. And it is obviously a great shame because through our scientific work we could make available a large amount of data and knowledge which would be of great benefit to WADA. But they are not interested.[35]

If it is true that a highly qualified group of WADA-independent members of the scientific community has become disillusioned with the WADA science, how can arbitrators at the Court of Arbitration for Sport confidently judge athletes on the basis of that science? WADA Director David Howman explains in the same article that: 'The reason we have the rule of strict liability is to protect the right of clean athletes.' But if anti-doping science is substandard, this argument is untenable. It does not strengthen the trust in the system that Howman shrugs off the substantial scientific criticism by taking the boldest relativistic position:

> [Howman:] We listen to our critics. [. . .] We are totally open [but] occasionally I have to declare that I disagree with people – especially with scientists. Globally it is difficult to find scientists who agree 100 percent. One of the reasons they are scientists is that they want to debate. This is what they get their money for. [. . .] There will always be some scientists who disagree with others. It's healthy.
>
> [Interviewer:] In the scientific world there is something which is more true than other?
>
> [Howman:] There you are wrong. I am not a scientist, but I have had to do with many scientists with many different opinions.[36]

If Howman means what he says, it is not immediately clear how he can have faith in the operation he is managing. If those scientists who say anti-doping testing is unreliable are neither closer nor farther from the truth than those scientists who say doping controls are reliable, it would be disconcerting if truth and reliability were alpha and omega in anti-doping. But this would also be a naïve assumption.

The Adverse Effect of Institutional Loyalty

The reason why Howman can be unalarmed, despite his relativistic perception of science, is that anti-doping is not primarily about developing a flawless test system, but about preservations of power and control over sport. As manifested in the film *The War on Doping* (2012), which featured commentary from Howman and Saugy among many others, anti-doping is perceived by many of its advocates as a *war* against drug use in sport.

To win that war, you must use power and testing is a powerful weapon. It may not be the most reliable weapon as it may often miss the target (false negatives) and accidentally hit innocent people (false positives), but so long as it puts the heat on the opposition it is functional. Hence, those who hold this view will be inclined to regard critics of any anti-doping measure as being in alliance with the opponents. Whether the critics actively want to harm the anti-doping campaign or it is their scientific conscience that makes them protest makes little difference. In any case, the critics are on the wrong side of things and ought to keep quiet as Sottas' et al. instructed *Nature*'s editor-in-chief.

When the weapons at hand prove insufficient, the situation becomes increasingly critical. Accepting defeat is not an option. Therefore, anti-doping campaigners call for additional and stronger measures. Initially, anti-doping tests were only carried out in competition and athletes were allowed to produce urine samples behind closed doors. However, revelations of athletes cheating during this procedure led to the rule that athletes should produce the sample in the presence of control officers. This humiliating demand has caused athletes to suffer from painful inability to urinate during doping controls.[37] Still cheating took place. When it became harder to fool the control, the doping practice changed. Some athletes continued to take advantage of banned drugs when they prepared for competitions. They just stopped treatment in time to be clean in competition. As a countermeasure, the IOC introduced out-of-competition controls in 1994.[38] This new weapon prompted doping athletes to hide away when they were doping. Thus, for out-of-competition to have any effect, it was necessary to oblige athletes to submit whereabouts information. This rule was introduced by WADA in 2003. But even with this far-reaching surveillance programme in place, doping continued. A major problem was that a number of efficient performance-enhancing drugs – not to mention blood transfusion – were undetectable in urine. In order to close that gap, some of the most doping-tarnished sports had already introduced blood profiling to supplement the urine testing in 1997. Various police raids and retired athletes' testimony revealed that this was to little avail as well. Despite blood testing and the development of the biological passport programme, the use of doping was still rife. So in 2010, the UCI made it compulsory for all Pro-Tour cyclist to participate in the UCI's biological passport programme.[39]

The ordinary doping controls impotence made it clear that if anti-doping should be remotely successful, it needed new flanks. Hence in 2010 during the preparation for the 2012 Olympics, UK Anti-doping opened a confidential hotline where people who became aware of or had reasoned suspicion of doping could safely pass on this information to the UK Anti-doping Intelligence Unit. Encouraged by the exposure and confessions of Lance

Armstrong which was a result of Federal Agent Jeff Novitzky's investigation of possible misuse of Federal money within the US Postal cycling team, WADA is now promoting the idea of closer collaboration between law enforcement and anti-doping organisations.[40] One can only speculate how prominent interrogation and intelligence work will be in the fight against doping in the future. At any rate, it is logical that the more weapons the anti-doping authorities store in their armoury, the bigger the risk of power abuse.

When anti-doping was limited to urine testing, clean athletes' only fears were of a false positive test or positive tests through unintentional – or in WADA terms: negligent – ingestion of a banned product. An unknown number of athletes have had their career terminated or severely damaged by such accidents. The reason why we do not know the extent of this is that guilty athletes may also protest their innocence by asserting that they were victims of unintentional doping in an attempt to get off the hook. Proving intent is obviously very difficult, even for scientists, thus determining whether an adverse analytical finding is indeed a true case of food contamination or a false positive remained vexing.

However, in some cases such as the British alpine skier Alain Baxter's, there is no doubt that his positive test had nothing to do with cheating or negligence in any meaningful sense of the word. Even so he had to forfeit the bronze medal he won in the slalom at the 2002 Olympics in Salt Lake City. Baxter had used a Vicks Vapor inhaler purchased in Utah apparently identical to the inhalers he usually bought in Britain to treat his chronic nasal congestion. What he could not have anticipated was that his inhalers were different in one crucial way. The American version contained traces of a methamphetamine-like chemical. Despite a Vicks scientist testifying that the chemical did not have methamphetamine's stimulating effect, an arbitration panel ruled that because the chemicals had a similar structure, Baxter was guilty.[41] If suspects of doping regulation infringements were admitted due process or if the burden of proof rested on WADA to prove the athlete had received any benefit, there is little doubt Baxter would have been acquitted. The problem is, however, that many other doping cases tried in a proper court would not have resulted in a ban either.

The Vulnerability of Athletes Exemplified by the Controversial Cases of Alberto Contador and Claudia Pechstein

A prominent example of the dilemma is the Spanish cyclist Alberto Contador's positive test for a minuscule amount (50 pg/ml) of the peptide hormone clenbuterol. The quantity found in his sample provided on July 21, 2010 during the Tour de France was 400 times below the amount that a WADA-accredited laboratory must be able to detect.[42] Contador's tests provided earlier in the race had all been negative. Thus, it is unlikely that he should have used the hormone to any effect during the race. Contador claimed that he must have been a victim of food contamination suggesting that he got the hormone in his system by eating a steak. The Spanish Cycling Federation's disciplinary committee accepted this possibility and acquitted him. However, both the UCI and the WADA contested this decision by appeal to CAS and, on February 6, 2012, the arbitrators set aside the Spanish ruling of February 14, 2011.

CAS emphasised in its Arbitral Award that in the event of an adverse analytical finding, the burden of proof rests with the athlete. Contador's team had not managed to convince the arbitrators that the Clenbuterol's route of entry into Contador's body was more likely to have happened than not have happened, that it was more likely than any other explanation as for instance by a contaminated food supplement or blood transfusion and that Contador had not been negligent.[43]

Contador still insists that he was banned for eating contaminated meat. Whatever the truth is, this case is yet another proof that the legal protection of athletes accused of doping is very limited. This is a serious enough issue in itself but it is clear that with the addition of weapons, and the presumption of guilt which underpins anti-doping testing, the vulnerability of the athletes increases.

A grave example is the 2-year suspension of German speed skater Claudia Pechstein in 2009. The five-time Olympic gold medallist was banned on the basis of her biological blood profile monitored by the International Skating Union. Pechstein had submitted blood samples for this programme from February 4, 2000 to April 30, 2009.[44] During those 9 years, she underwent numerous in and out-of-competition controls. None of these controls resulted in an adverse analytical finding but her blood profile had been atypical. According to the International Skating Union (ISU), 0.4–2.4% reticulocytes are considered the normal range. However, some of Pechstein's tests had been 'well above the value of 2.4 per cent followed by sharp decrease'.[45] Her deviant blood profile combined with her outstanding performances made her a natural suspect of doping. When she was tested on February 6, 2009, the day before the beginning of the ISU World Championships, she submitted a blood sample. Her reticulocytes count was measured at 3.49%. In the eyes of the ISU responsible, this was too high not to be a case of 'doping'. Because of this abnormal test result, she was retested on the February 7, 2009 in the morning and in the afternoon. These samples showed 3.54% and 3.38% reticulocytes, respectively.[46] Despite her haemoglobin and haematocrit levels were below the 'no-start' threshold, the German Speed Skating Union decided to withdraw Pechstein from the event after consultation with ISU medical advisor Dr Harm Kuipers. A little more than a week later, Pechstein had a new blood test taken once again showing a sharp decrease in reticulocytes. This time, it was measured at 1.37%.

After reviewing Pechstein's blood profile, ISU filed a statement of complaint with the ISU Disciplinary Commission, which resulted in a two-year suspension with the aver that Pechstein was guilty of blood doping. Pechstein appealed to CAS.

In her defence, Pechstein drew attention to the fact that the ISU biological passport programme did not follow the WADA guidelines. If her blood profile had been accessed in accordance with these guidelines, there would have never been a case in the first place. The arbitrational panel disregarded Pechstein's

> contention that the WADA Draft Biological Passport Guidelines should be followed by the ISU as "minimum standards" because, as correctly pointed out by the ISU, that document is a draft which has not been finalized yet and which will not be mandatory even when it is eventually adopted.[47]

It is true that the WADA's guidelines were yet to be finalised when the arbitrators were hearing the case. The guidelines were only finalised a week after CAS published its verdict which upheld the ISU ruling. But it is also true that these scientific-based guidelines had been developed and negotiated years before. In other words, the draft circulated did not consist of an unsubstantiated non-committal set of ideas. So the arbitrators could have assessed the WADA draft, which proposed a 99.9% probability in contrast to the ISU 95.0 threshold of per cent probability. Had the arbitrators considered the background for this discrepancy, they might have come to a different conclusion. At least they would have understood that the statistical risk of an innocent athlete potentially being sanctioned would be 1 in 20 athletes following the ISU programme whereas the WADA draft guidelines, now officially in place, warranted that statistically only 1 in 1000 athletes will be a false positive.

It should be noted that an athlete is not automatically sanctioned on the basis of the blood values. When a suspicious blood profile is observed, an expert panel assesses the case before a case is opened, and this procedure means that the risk of a false conviction under both the ISU and the WADA guidelines are less than 1 in 20 athletes or 1 in 1000 athletes, respectively. But having said that, it should also be noted that the same experts supporting biological passports as an indirect doping test might also be asked to later interpret any abnormal findings. So how much extra protection the expert evaluation gives is dubious considering their conflicting interests.

At any rate, Pechstein's conviction inspired once again a number of independent scientists to criticise anti-doping. This time, the target was the science behind the biological passport.[48] From a scientific point of view, the blood profile did not make any sense. Reticulocytes are immature red blood cells. Typically, an elevated number of reticulocytes are found in athletes treated with EPO in the boosting period. The immature red blood cells are unable to carry oxygen. So if Pechstein had been using EPO during her preparation for the World Championships, she had got it utterly wrong. She would not have had any benefit from the EPO injections because the blood cells would not have matured until after the event had taken place. Even more, she would have been more likely to test positive for EPO in-competition. For that reason, no experienced or well-advised athlete would use high dosages of EPO shortly before competing. If such an athlete would use EPO doping the athlete would either take EPO weeks before competition to allow the reticulocytes to mature and the EPO to clear the system, use micro dosages, which do not critically impact the blood profile of an athlete or use autologous blood transfusions, which has the opposite effect of high dosages of EPO in that it decreases the reticulocytes count. In light of this, independent experts found it hard to believe that Pechstein had indeed doped.[49] Nevertheless, on the basis of the scientific evidence provided, the arbitrators concluded:

> that the abnormal values of [reticulocytes] recorded on 18 February 2009, cannot be reasonably explained by any congenital or subsequently developed abnormality. The Panel finds that they must therefore derive from the Athlete's illicit manipulation of her own blood, which remains the only reasonable alternative source of such abnormal values.[50]

Considering the novelty of the biological passport and that it was utilised as an indirect doping-detection method without any causal connection proven, it could be expected that the arbitration panel would require a higher degree of certainty that Pechstein's blood profile was caused by doping than what the ISU guidelines warrant.

The CAS set-up is arranged so that the athletes cannot appoint their favoured defence lawyer to sit on the panel. They must choose their representative from a fixed list of arbitrators, who by inclusion in this list have accepted the CAS principles, which give the athletes less protection than they would have in an ordinary court. By accepting these principles, the arbitrators have in effect sided with sports' governing bodies. This leaves the athletes disadvantaged. In relation to this particular case, it invites speculation that the arbitrators have sought to protect the anti-doping authorities' new anti-doping weapon – the biological passport – rather than serve the ideal of justice.

Further disconcerting is once again the reaction to criticism from those who have stock in the biological passport. An uncompromising critic of the biological passport programme, the Dutch chemometrician Klaas Faber, who wrote an expert opinion in favour of Pechstein, insisted that the biological passport was based on flawed statistics. He contacted WADA's Medical Director, Dr Rabin, and informed him about his views, leaving little doubt that he thought Pechstein was a victim of a miscarriage of justice. This possibility did not seem to bother Rabin who responded that 'Mrs Pechstein's case was not reviewed under the Athletes Passport model as developed by WADA, but under the ISU longitudinal model. Not the same rules and not the same science in support'.[51] In other words, Rabin conceded that Pechstein's doping sanction was based on a science unapproved by WADA. Nevertheless, the organisation – purportedly fighting for fair play for clean athletes – did not voice any concern that Pechstein could be unjustly convicted on the basis of the unsafe ISU guidelines.

The suspicion that Pechstein was sacrificed to promote the biological passport only grew when Dr Sottas, who developed the athletes' passport model, admitted in a statement published on September 29, 2010 that 'it is not possible to analyse the blood data of Mrs Pechstein with the model I have developed simply because the collection, transport and analysis of the blood samples did not follow the corresponding WADA protocols'.[52] Sottas did not offer this information when he received the data on February 12, 2009, a week after the ISU World Championships. It is beyond Faber why 'Dr Sottas rated the single indirect evidence incriminating Claudia Pechstein in a manner that largely contradicts his own work on the biological passport'.[53] However, Sottas' initial reluctance to dismiss the ISU data is not incomprehensible with the concept 'corrupt idealism' in mind.

The reason why Sottas and others worked to develop the biological passport programme was to improve the anti-doping system so that fewer athletes could get away with doping. Their goal was to catch the doping cheats. Pechstein had had an outstanding career winning her first Olympic gold medal in 1994, during the EPO heydays, and her last in Turin 2006, when blood doping scandals were exposed in Spain and Austria. She might be the exact kind of athlete the biological passport was designed to detect. When Sottas received Pechstein's test results from the ISU and was asked to assess her blood profile, he confirmed unequivocally that her profile was abnormal, disregarding the fact that her profile was within the limits of the WADA guidelines. By doing so, he encouraged the ISU to use his model to prosecute Pechstein. Yet Sottas subsequently stated in an interview that he had informed the ISU that Pechstein's profile was not a typical doping profile.[54] This indicates that he was not entirely comfortable with the conviction after all. However, the fact that Sottas did not turn out to defend Pechstein before the CAS had passed sentence suggests that he prioritised the promotion of the new weapon in the fight against doping over the protection of an athlete against a potentially false conviction.

Conclusion

Since anti-doping testing was introduced in cycling in 1965, the anti-doping campaign has developed dramatically. Until the formation of WADA in 1999, doping regulations, tests and sanctions were the various sports' own businesses. In most sports, sanctions were relatively mild. Previous doping violations could be as little as two-week suspension.[55] It speaks volumes of the changes WADA has spurred that riders who were excluded from the Tour de France 1998 after being found guilty of systematic EPO doping were welcomed back in the race in 1999. One of those riders, Alex Zülle who was arrested and during interrogation admitted to doping since 1993, was even celebrated on the podium as he managed to finish second overall after Lance Armstrong.

The history of doping shows that a soft educational approach to drugs in sport is unavailing. A far-reaching and uncompromising regime is required if anti-doping shall have any real impact. To influence public opinion and convince politicians that doping infringement is more serious than other forms of cheating in sport, idealistic anti-doping pioneers have not shied away from fabrication or exaggeration of stories about the devastating effects of performance-enhancing drugs, as this study has shown. Anti-doping idealists have successfully lobbied for harsher penalties and stronger anti-doping measures. As a consequence, it has become much more serious to be found guilty of a doping offence.

For professional athletes, a first-time offence takes away their livelihood for a couple of years and is potentially career ending. In effect, doping infringements have become pseudo-criminal in nature.[56] Hence, the foundation for the claim that doping is a sport rule infringement and thus should be tried in sports' own legal system without possibility to appeal is eroding. The lack of transparency in anti-doping science, the hostility towards scientific criticism, the dubious convictions of a number of athletes and the absolute power of the sports governing bodies notwithstanding the formal separation of powers between the sports organisations, WADA and CAS are indicative of a self-sufficient and unreliable system. So if anti-doping cases cannot be transferred to an ordinary legal system with proper checks and balances without dismantling anti-doping, an independent body financed by the athletes union to watch the work of the anti-doping authorities ought to be considered a proper alternative. Since the rules are meant to serve and protect the interests of the athletes, it is hard to understand why they should not have a say in the development and administration of the rules. In fact, to paraphrase Rousseau, they ought to be their author.

Notes on Contributor

Verner Møller, is Professor of Sport and Body Culture at Aarhus University, Denmark. His main research interests are elite sport and body cultural extremes. He has published a number of books and articles on doping and is co-founder of the International Network of Humanistic Doping Research.

Notes

1. Christiansen and Møller, *Mål medicin og moral* and Hanstad and Loland, "Elite Athletes' Duty."
2. Palmer and Baer-Hoffmann, "WADA Code Review."
3. Ibid., 4.
4. Ibid., 5.
5. Death Penalty Information Center, "The Innocent List."
6. Pound, *Inside the Olympics*, 272.
7. Vinton, N. "As New Alpine Season Begins, Miller Makes Himself Heard Again" (*The New York Times*, October 23, 2005). http://www.nytimes.com/2005/10/23/sports/othersports/23ski.html?n=Top%2FReference%2FTimes%20Topics%2FPeople%2FM%2FMiller%2C%20Bode&_r = 0.
8. "Bode Miller's Take On Doping In Alpine Skiing: Legalize It?" (*Ski Racing Magazine*, 2005). http://skiracing.com/?q=node/2998.
9. "WADA Chief Criticizes Miller's Doping Comments" (*Associated Press,* 2005). http://sports.espn.go.com/oly/news/story?id=2203195.
10. IOC, Ethics Commission, "Decision with Recommendation No. D07/01."
11. Hart, S. "Dick Pound: Making Enemies was Part of Job" (*The Telegraph*, November 11, 2007). http://www.telegraph.co.uk/sport/othersports/drugsinsport/2325475/Dick-Pound-Making-enemies-was-part-of-job.html.
12. "Apologise, Mr Pound" (*Jamaica Observer*, August 17, 2012). http://www.jamaicaobserver.com/editorial/Apologise–Mr-Pound.
13. Wivel, K. "WADA: Lukkede circler [WADA: Closed Circles]" (*Weekendavisen*, April 23, 2010).
14. Møller, *The Scapegoat.*
15. Rousseau, *The Social Contract*, 4.
16. Ibid., 41.
17. Dimeo, *A History of Drug Use.*
18. Ibid.
19. Ibid.
20. Møller, "Knud Enemark Jensen's Death."
21. Bøgeskov, L. "Doping-mysteriet uden løsning [The Doping Mystery Without Solution]" (*Politiken –Sportsmagasinet*, April 9, 2001, 12).

22. López, "'Drug of Mass Destruction'," 87.
23. Ibid., 96.
24. Ibid.
25. Ibid.
26. Banfi et al., "A World Apart," 1007.
27. Berry, "The Science of Doping."
28. Ibid.
29. Nature, "A Level Playing Field."
30. Sottas, Saudan, and Saugy, "Doping."
31. Ibid.
32. Lundby et al., "Testing for Recombinant Human Erythropoietin," 417.
33. Saugy, Robinson, and Lamon, "To the Editor."
34. Ibid.
35. Wivel, K. "WADA: Lukkede circler [WADA: Closed Circles]" (*Weekendavisen*, April 23, 2010).
36. Ibid.
37. Elbe, Schlegel, and Brand "Psychogenic Urine Retention"
38. Patrick, "Passport to Clean Competition."
39. Ibid.
40. WADA, "Intelligence Experts Emphasize Importance."
41. Hiltzik, M. "Athletes' Unbeatable Foe" (*Los Angeles Times*, December 10, 2006). http://articles.latimes.com/2006/dec/10/sports/sp-doping10.
42. CAS, "CAS 2011/A/2384 UCI v. Alberto Contador Velasco & RFEC."
43. Ibid.
44. CAS, "CAS 2009/A/1912 Claudia Pechstein v/International Skating Union."
45. Ibid.
46. Ibid.
47. Ibid., 30.
48. Hellmann, F. "Interview mit Anti-Doping-Experten: 'Pechstein past nicht in ein Epo-Profil'" (*Frankfurter Rundschau*, *Sport*, November 30, 2009).
49. Ibid.
50. CAS, "CAS 2009/A/1912 Claudia Pechstein v/International Skating Union," 60.
51. Faber, "The Strange Case."
52. Ibid.
53. Ibid.
54. Geisser, R. "Die überhörten Zweifel [The Unheard Doubt]" (*Neue Zürcher Zeitung*, March 27, 2010).
55. Dimeo, *A History of Drug Use*.
56. Soek, *The Strict Liability Principles*.

References

Banfi, G., G. Lombardi, A. Colombini, and G. Lippi. "A World Apart – Inaccuracies of Laboratory Methodologies in Antidoping Testing." *Clinica Chimica Acta* 411 (2010): 1003–1008.

Berry, D. A. "The Science of Doping." *Nature* 454, no. 7 (2008): 692–693.

CAS. "CAS 2009/A/1912 Claudia Pechstein v/International Skating Union. CAS 2009/A/1913 Deutsche Eisschnelllauf Gemeinschaft e-V. v/International Skating Union." 2009. http://www.tas-cas.org/d2wfiles/document/3802/5048/0/FINAL20AWARD20PECHSTEIN.pdf

CAS. "CAS 2011/A/2384 UCI v. Alberto Contador Velasco & RFEC," 2012. Accessed February 11, 2013. http://www.tas-cas.org/d2wfiles/document/5648/5048/0/FINAL20AWARD202012.02.06.pdf

Christiansen, A. V., and V. Møller. *Mål medicin og moral – om eliteatleters opfattelse af sport, doping og fairplay* [Goals, Medicine and Moral]. Odense: University of Southern Denmark Press, 2007.

Death Penalty Information Center. "The Innocent List." 2012. http://www.deathpenaltyinfo.org/innocence-list-those-freed-death-row

Dimeo, P. *A History of Drug Use in Sport 1876–1976*. London: Routledge, 2007.

Elbe, A.-M., M. M. Schlegel, and R. Brand. "Psychogenic Urine Retention During Doping Controls: Consequences for Elite Athletes." *Performance Enhancement & Health* 1 (2012): 66–74.

Faber, K. "The Strange Case of Dr Sottas and Mr Hyde – Why Would Anyone Withhold Claudia Pechstein Decisive Exonerating Evidence?" 2010. http://sottas.info

Hanstad, D. V., and S. Loland. "Elite Athletes' Duty to Provide Information on Their Whereabouts: Justifiable Anti-doping Work or an Indefensible Surveillance Regime?" *European Journal of Sport Science* 9, no. 1 (2009): 3–10.

IOC, Ethics Commission. "Decision with Recommendation No. D07/01." 2007. http://www.olympic.org/Documents/Reports/EN/en_report_1127.pdf

Jelkmann, W. E. "Testing for Recombinant Human Erythropoietin – The Bouquets of Compounds." *Journal of Applied Physiology* 105, no. 6 (2008): 1992–1993.

López, B. "The Invention of a 'Drug of Mass Destruction': Deconstructing the EPO Myth." *Sport in History* 31, no. 1 (2011): 84–109.

Lundby, C., N. J. Achman-Andersen, J. J. Thomsen, A. M. Nørgaard, and P. Robach. "Testing for Recombinant Human Erythropoietin in Urine: Problems Associated with Current Anti-doping Testing." *Journal of Applied Physiology* 105 (2008): 417–419.

Møller, V. "Knud Enemark Jensen's Death During the Rome Olympics 1960 – A Search for Truth?" *Sport in History* 25, no. 3 (2005): 452–471.

Møller, V. *The Scapegoat – About the Expulsion of Michael Rasmussen from the Tour de France 2007 and Beyond*. Copenhagen: People's Press, 2011.

Nature, "A Level Playing Field." *Nature* 454 (2008): 667. doi:10.1038/454667a.

Palmer, W., and J. Baer-Hoffmann. "'WADA Code Review' First Submission March 15, 2012." http://antidopingreform.files.wordpress.com/2012/03/finaldraftwadarevision-5.pdf

Patrick, K. "Passport to Clean Competition." *British Medical Journal* 344 (2012): e2077.

Pound, D. *Inside the Olympics*. Toronto: Wiley, 2004.

Rousseau, J.-J. *The Social Contract*. New York: Barnes and Noble, 2005.

Saugy, M., N. Robinson, and S. Lamon. "To the Editor." *Journal of Applied Physiology* 105, no. 2 (2008): 417–419.

Soek, J.-W. *The Strict Liability Principles and the Human Rights of Athletes in Doping Cases*. Den Haag: T.M.C. Asser.

Sottas, P., C. Saudan, and M. Saugy. "Doping: A Paradigm Shift Has Taken Place in Testing." *Nature* 455 (2008): 166. doi:10.1038/455166a.

WADA. "Intelligence Experts Emphasize Importance of Legislation and Information Sharing." 2013. http://playtrue.wada-ama.org/news/intelligence-experts-emphasize-the-importance-of-legislation-and-information-sharing/

Why Lance Armstrong? Historical Context and Key Turning Points in the 'Cleaning Up' of Professional Cycling

Paul Dimeo

School of Sport, University of Stirling, Stirling, UK

The US Anti-Doping Agency published its evidence against Lance Armstrong in October 2012 after a lengthy investigation and a series of testimonies from his former US Postal Service teammates. This article aims to understand the development processes – local and global – that led eventually to his 'confession' in January 2013 on the Oprah Winfrey show. By taking a chronological approach from the 1980s onwards, the following key themes will be addressed: the doping state of play when Armstrong began his career; the incremental confessions of other cyclists that helped break down cycling's secret doping culture; the broader organisational changes in anti-doping; the reasons why Armstrong became the focal point of anti-doping efforts; and the implications for professional cycling and anti-doping in the near future. Thus, the aim is to synthesise macro- and micro-level developments to explain the outcomes, and to further understand the consequences of this 'scandal'.

Introduction

There is no doubt that 2012 was a memorable year for international sports. The London Olympics and Paralympics was a good news story of a well-planned event and dramatic spectacles. However, the more interesting story of the year – which provoked debate from experts and onlookers – was the public humiliation of arguably the most triumphant sportsman of the twenty-first century, Lance Armstrong. When the US Anti-Doping Agency (USADA) released its detailed report of the evidence gathered against him,[1] the story was international headline news. When he famously appeared on the Oprah Winfrey show to 'confess' to what had been alleged, the national and international viewing figures totalled 28 million across 190 countries and was broadcast in 30 languages.[2]

The discussions of Armstrong's fall from grace are wide-ranging, and can be found in mainstream media, cycling publications, online public forums such as blogs and in the writings of investigative journalists who helped to uncover the details of the case.[3] These have covered political, ethical and legal issues. The former have asked questions of failings in the leadership and policies over the past years that allowed doping to continue unabated despite the rhetoric of anti-doping ideology. The ethical debate has led to critical and at times angry judgements made against Armstrong, his teammates, his doctors and the media. The legal issues have focused upon the nature of the evidence, how it was collected and whether his rights for representation have been respected through the Court of Arbitration process. The consequences of law suits to reclaim sponsorship and prize money have yet to be resolved.[4] Yet the outcome is clear, by choosing not to defend the case through arbitration, Armstrong has allowed the decision to be accepted and his sanctions include a life-time ban and the stripping of his titles.[5]

This article begins by considering the state of doping culture in cycling when Armstrong arrived on the scene in the mid-1990s.[6] Essentially, there was a choice facing any aspiring professional rider, which was to take banned drugs or be at a competitive disadvantage.[7] The failings of anti-doping to 'level the playing field' are evident in the number of tests Armstrong and other riders 'passed', and in the confidence sports doctors had in planning dosages in such a way as to circumvent the testing system.[8] The period of success in Armstrong's career therefore can best be understood as belonging to the era of doping. By 2005, when he retired as seven-time winner of the Tour de France and the sport's most illustrious champion, the era of doping was gradually beginning to give way to the pressures of anti-doping, notably the development of a global approach through the World Anti-Doping Agency (WADA). The second part of the article examines the internal and external developments that gradually lent authority to anti-doping agencies and which eroded the *omerta* that had protected doping cyclists from outsiders. When Armstrong came out of retirement in 2009 and also competed in marathons, mountain biking events and triathlons, anti-doping had been empowered by events in cycling and other sports. The allegations that emerged against him were investigated by a Federal commission in the USA and then by USADA. Thus, the body of evidence left him nowhere to turn but a public ritual of confession in the hope of returning to sport. The final sections of the article ask questions about why Armstrong was the focus of such a sustained anti-doping effort, and the policy implications going forward of the procedures and processes underlying this apparent victory for anti-doping and the supposedly successful 'cleaning-up' of professional cycling.

The overarching objective therefore is to track the various events – planned and unplanned – which explain how Lance Armstrong, who began his career in the era of doping, was finally defeated by the rising power of anti-doping, and to consider the ongoing implications for anti-doping policy.

The 1980s and 1990s: An Open Field for Doping

When Lance Armstrong began his attempt to conquer professional cycling, doping was commonplace and cyclists had constructed an *omerta*, or code of silence.[9] In the 1990s, this was a niche sport, dominated by Europeans, lacking worldwide media coverage and lacking any systematic effort to tackle doping which was tacitly tolerated by the spectators. The international fight against doping was a fragmented affair: the International Olympic Committee was providing some leadership but focused mainly on the quadrennial Games and lacked any significant influence on professional cycling. The testing system varied across sport and place, such that some competitors were rarely tested and most sports only focused on in-competition testing, allowing dopers free rein to consume banned drugs during their training periods. Investigative journalists, such as David Walsh who would become famous for making accusations against Lance Armstrong, did little to expose doping. Walsh writes that he strongly suspected Irishman Sean Kelly in the mid-1980s; he rationalised that he was not really cheating given the wider context of the demands of professional cycling, and in fact it was not until the rumours about Lance Armstrong and small pieces of evidence against him emerged that Walsh took doping seriously as a public interest story.[10] The testing system was so lax that cyclists felt confident of beating it.[11] There was little by way of out-of-competition testing, and a lack of stringent application of regulations. With the support of professional team managers and unscrupulous doctors, cyclists could use new substances and techniques and stay ahead of the testers. The Scottish cyclist Graeme Obree said in 1996 that he thought 99% of elite-level riders were using erythropoietin (EPO) 'to be at the same level as the others'. He himself spoke openly later about his decision not to dope and thus sacrificing potential career advancement:

> I still feel I was robbed of part of my career. I was signed up to ride in the prologue of the Tour back in 1995, but it was made very obvious to me I would have to take drugs. I said no, no way, and I was sacked by my team ... I feel I was robbed by a lot of these bastards taking drugs.[12]

The President of the Union Cycliste Internationale (UCI), Hein Verbruggen, admitted the authorities could not keep up with the new drugs used by cyclists and that attempts to control doping were 'ineffective'.[13] Fifteen years later, the American professional cyclist Tyler Hamilton, who had been a teammate of Lance Armstrong, described in some amusing detail the strategies for avoiding testers such as giving vague whereabouts information, not answering the door when they called, getting others to lie for him and (in collusion with the team doctor) abusing the Therapeutic Use Exemption system to take substances like cortisone.[14]

The evidence of doping across three decades is increasingly mounting and we are finding out more with each new confession.[15] Møller writes that prior to the late 1990s,

> teams had an astonishingly easy-going attitude to doping substances ... and did not do much to keep what was going on under wraps. Used needles and syringes were dumped in public rubbish containers or thrown in rubbish bags in the teams' hotel rooms.[16]

However, few within or indeed outside the sport were determined to confront the issue, that was until the most controversial revelations came during the 1998 Tour de France, when the Festina team were caught by border police with a large array of doping products including EPO, growth hormone and synthetic testosterone.[17] Later evidence showed that the team's doctor flushed tens of thousands of dollars of performance-enhancing drugs down the toilet of the team's camper during the race.[18]

The extent of doping within that team, the subsequent discovery of doping within other teams and the detailed revelations from those who confessed demonstrate the full extent of the problem through the 1990s and early 2000s. As John Hoberman explained of this time period, professional cycling was:

> A celebrated subculture whose drug-taking was quietly tolerated, as political authorities and the general public chose not to address the consumption of drugs within this milieu .... The solidarity of the professional cycling fraternity has accommodated the clandestine consumption of illicit drugs.[19]

While the Festina scandal was lauded as a potential turning point for anti-doping investigations, what it really showed was that doping controls 'were useless or even fraudulent'.[20] More so, the attitudes of the cyclists themselves suggested a tolerant view of doping, much like in a previous era when Jacques Anquetil proclaimed that professionals should be allowed to use drugs. The participants of the 1998 Tour, protested by 'downing the tools of their trade (i.e. their bikes and bodies) and "striking" ... because of the police and the press, who each in their own way supported the anti-doping initiative'.[21] The few riders who spoke out against doping found themselves ostracised by the peloton. This apparent seismic shock did little to deter dopers: the Scottish rider David Millar recalls how other riders in the peloton were surprised by the anti-doping stance he took during his early incursions in the Grand Tours from 2000 onwards.[22]

The witness testimony provided in USADA's 'Reasoned Decision' statement shows that Lance Armstrong had decided to use performance-enhancing drugs before 1998, though he was not a competitor in that year's Tour de France. Jonathan Vaughters was a teammate of Armstrong in 1998 and explained how both of them used EPO during that season.[23] However, what is interesting for setting the historical context of Armstrong and others' decision to dope was the lack of proper doping controls and the sense that without 'medical support' they could not compete at the highest levels of their chosen sport – the choice was to stay and play dirty or go home clean. That moment of truth, as it were, came a few years previously:

> In 1994, Armstrong's second season as a professional did not match the excellence of his first. The abuse of EPO, a new performance enhancing wonder drug, was spreading in the peloton and Armstrong struggled to compete in the early season classics. In July, on the eve of his second Tour de France, he alluded to the changes in an interview with the journalist, Samuel Abt. 'It's harder to race this year, cycling is harder now. In a year, I tell you, man. I hate to point fingers, and I'm not going to do that. But there are a lot of guys who are a lot better and a lot faster than last year'.[24]

This is not to say Armstrong was ever determined to stay clean, or that he had a strong moral dissatisfaction with the prospect of doping. A number of riders, who were either caught or voluntarily confessed, portray themselves as idealists gradually worn down by a repressive culture that leaves them nowhere to turn but into the arms of a doctor whose comforting words relieve the protagonist of their guilt while the fresh blood or the drugs are pumping through their system. Armstrong's descent into doping seems to be upfront, emotional, vigorous and realistic in its acceptance of his own decision-making capabilities, at least as described by Frankie Andreu, a teammate and mentor, reflecting on the 1994 season:

> The thing about Lance was he had to be successful, he didn't want a career that was average. At this time the whole thing bugged him, it ate into him. He would bitch about it all the time, 'This is bullshit ... these guys are flying ... I can't believe he's doing this... I should be killing these guys.' He did not say, 'I am going to get on a program,' he never said anything like that, but, man, he was frustrated, and I am sure it was as a result of that he decided to begin working with (the doping expert) Michele Ferrari.[25]

One of the most famous stories to come out of the USADA inquiry relates to a moment during Armstrong's cancer treatment in October 1996. Several witnesses testified that when asked by doctors in an Indiana hospital whether he had used any performance-enhancing drugs, he admitted the use of EPO, testosterone, human growth hormone, steroids and cortisone.[26] So we can assume that Armstrong was intimate with the doping culture of the mid-1990s, then continued his usage during the highly successful phase of his career 1999–2005. The evidence gathered and presented by USADA would support this. What becomes of interest is the gradual erosion of the *omerta*, the incremental strengthening of anti-doping and the important turning points that led eventually to his demise. In the space of a decade, the acceptance of doping, or least the view that cyclists should be left alone to make their own decisions, had more or less disappeared. Part of the reason for this relates to the expanding resources and reach of anti-doping supported by a series of investigative journalists on the hunt for good stories. However, part of the reason lies with the doping revelations from cyclists themselves, insider accounts gradually building up to a crescendo over the 2000–2010 decade, which no longer could be excused away by cycling's leadership as 'rotten apples'. And thus, even before USADA amassed its evidence against Armstrong, it was argued that 'the gentle trickle of revelations is slowly making the general public somewhat accustomed to the thought that doping is part of the reality of sport, [and] it is apparently not prepared to accept it'.[27] This change in perceptions is recent. The doping cases of 2004–2005 in cycling did not register much media attention beyond cycling.[28] Even in 2009, the *Guardian* writer and author Lawrence Donegan claimed that the 'public doesn't care about athletes taking drugs'.[29] Indeed, when David Walsh of the *Sunday Times* was interviewing Armstrong's former teammates and associated people such as Besty Andreu through the early 2000s, he came to realise that he was probably the only person trying to find evidence about Armstrong and doping.[30] Thus, the rising interest can be attributed in some ways to the determination of anti-doping authorities and the series of cyclists who detailed the doping culture. However, the wider public interest was also piqued by the bigger catch. Thus, the very biography and character of the 'villain', Lance Armstrong, the gradual sense that he would be found out and the drama of the chase, has made doping a news event once more.

The Power Shift towards Anti-Doping: Confessions and the Erosion of *Omerta*

One of the first professional cyclists to expose the culture of doping within the sport was the Irishman Paul Kimmage, who followed a career of sports writing after his athletic career was finished. However, he was intensely aware of the uniqueness of his position, and that deviating from the collective *omerta* was not considered acceptable by other riders:

> The law of silence: it exists not only in the Mafia but also in the peloton. Those who break the law, who talk to the press about the dope problems in the sport are despised. They are branded as having '*craché dans la soupe*', they have spat in the soup.[31]

Arguably, the beginning of this power shift was an accident: the discovery by border control officials in July 1998 of a vast array of doping products in the car of the Festina team's *soigneur*, Willy Voet. This was not a cycling investigation; however, the extent of doping revealed makes it hard to believe that cycling authorities did not suspect that some form of cheating was occurring, but instead left it to the French police to carry out the investigations. The events have been detailed elsewhere, not least in the book by Voet himself, which concludes with his pessimistic view of anti-doping's chances, despite the trauma of the 1998 Tour, and written in 1999:

> If nothing changes in the race between the drug-takers and the testers, the takers will always be a clear length ahead. Refrigerated lorries, magic suitcases, all these little secrets have been discovered. But other ways and means supplanted them. Unmarked cars waiting at cyclists' hotels, campervans full of fans which can travel anywhere with their fridges full of capsules hidden among the jampots, yoghurt and mozzarella. There are rumours that EPO will soon be detectable. What a result. EPO has already been overtaken by other methods of doping, based on reproducing cells and molecules.[32]

Such details were beginning to impress upon the public understanding of doping. Some of the top Festina riders had eventually confessed, and the team's director admitted that there was systematic doping within the team.

However, the strength of the *omerta*-related condemnation of outspoken anti-doping riders was illustrated in the difficulties faced by the Frenchman Christophe Bassons. When he questioned the claims made by cycling bodies that anti-doping was now more effective in the wake of Festina, he was ostracised by other professional riders. One example of intimidation came from Lance Armstrong, as Basson later reported:

> ... and then Lance Armstrong reached me. He grabbed my by the shoulder, because he knew that everyone would be watching, and he knew that at that moment, he could show everyone that he was the boss. He stopped me, and he said what I was saying wasn't true, what I was

> saying was bad for cycling, that I mustn't say it, that I had no right to be a professional cyclist, that I should quit cycling, that I should quit the tour, and finished by saying [*beep*] you ... I was depressed for 6 months. I was crying all of the time. I was in a really bad way.[33]

Basson's career and emotional well-being were severely damaged by the response to his anti-doping comments. Festina had not changed much about doping practices, but it had at least begun the process of revealing the nature of those practices. The fascination around Lance Armstrong's incredible story of returning from cancer to win the Tour de France was to bring more media and public attention to the sport. Armstrong himself benefited from this by publishing in 2001 an autobiography, *It's Not About the Bike: My Journey Back to Life*, which won the William Hill sports book of the year prize.

Further public criticisms of doping emerged from inside the sport from the early 2000s onwards. In March 2004, the Spanish rider, Jesús Manzano, provided details about the illegal practices conducted in the Kelme team, who had sacked him six months previously. The team management and doctors had colluded in blood doping of the riders in the 2003 season. As Christiansen writes,

> If we are to believe ... Manzano, the riders in the Spanish team [Kelme] have been more or less forced to take EPO and growth hormone, and they had to endure badly administered blood transfusions in connection with blood doping before the 2003 Tour de France.[34]

Around that same time there were a series of other doping scandals in cycling, including that the French team Cofidis 'had organized a major doping network' and that a doctor with the French Cycling Association said that 'at least 30 per cent of French riders were still using EPO'.[35]

A lesser known competitor, the American Matt DeCanio, has been campaigning against doping in cycling in the aftermath of his own experiences. He did not test positive during his career, but had ambivalent emotions regarding his time as a professional cyclist. He joined his first team in 1998 and told his story after retiring in 2003. He described in detail the doping practices of other cyclists, that many felt it was their right to do so, and the pressures placed upon him by the team managers. After resisting the pressure to dope for several years, he succumbed in 2003, but felt strongly that the wrong decision had been made. DeCanio has made several public statements about doping. Here is an extract from a longer account on his 'Stolen Underground' website:

> After the worlds in Italy where I placed 22nd place, I was asked to race for a U-23 team in Italy as I was considered the top racer of my generation by the Italians. This new team was a dream come true, racing in Florence, Italy and getting to see the world and to do my passion which was racing bicycles. I could not have been happier. But soon after arriving I realized that something was incredibly wrong with the events that were taking place. The first night I was there the riders were throwing needles at each other. All of my teammates were injecting themselves with various products and vitamins. I was scared, immature and I did not know what to do. None of my training at the United States Olympic Training Center had properly prepared me for the pressures I was now facing in Italy to inject myself. There was not a number to call or a single person to speak to about this. Later I would find out why this was the case. After the first season I would witness and speak to my teammates openly about doping. They all admitted to me other than 1 or 2 riders that they were using EPO and/or HGH. My managers all asked me to use these products and I refused which upset them and caused them to treat me less fairly than my other teammates. I was given a steel bicycle to race instead of an aluminum for example. I was not paid, and the other riders were paid. I was shunned by my teammates at dinner for my lacklustre performance while they were doping and winning. They would call me a loser. This all added up to a mental mind game that would forever affect me.[36]

A series of other confessions around this time served to publicly demonstrate that cycling's reputation was indeed true. A number of these were not motivated though by an ethical view that doping was cheating and the sport should be 'fair'. Instead, what we see is a murkier set of circumstances in which confessors often have something to gain by their new-found 'honesty'. One such case is the Scottish cyclist David Millar. He was the subject of a police investigation in which members of the Cofidis team were accused of doping in the early 2000s, and he was sanctioned to a two-year ban for EPO use in 2004. Once again, it was a criminal investigation rather than an internal cycling process that led to this outcome (many of the most important anti-doping successes have been by non-sports organisations). Millar was also unfortunate in that WADA had recently published the first version of the WADA Code which stated that a doping violation should result in a two-year ban. As Millar explained in interviews and in his autobiography, doping was part of the team's culture: eight others were charged in connection with the affair: Cédric Vasseur, Philippe Gaumont, Robert Sassone, Médéric Clain, Marek Rutkiewicz and Daniel Majewski (all riders), Boguslaw Madejak (ex-Cofidis physiotherapist) and Oleg Kozlitine (former *directeur sportif* of Oktos).[37]

Within a few years, other scandals rocked the sport. The death of Marco Pantani, winner of the 1998 Tour de France, brought details of his recreational and performance-enhancing drug use. *Operation Puerto* created a bizarre situation in which riders deemed under suspicion were not allowed to compete in the top races. The 2006 'winner' of the Tour, the American Floyd Landis, tested positive for testosterone and was disqualified. Michael Rasmussen was withdrawn from the 2007 Tour de France while wearing the yellow jersey and sacked by his team Rabobank for lying about his whereabouts despite not actually breaking any specific anti-doping regulations. He was subsequently banned for two years by the organisation that held his licence, the Monaco Cycling Federation from 2007–2009, and ban which was subsequently upheld by the Court of Arbitration for Sport (CAS).[38] The situation had descended into farce but slowly anti-doping policy-makers were gaining some ground on the doping culture in cycling.

However, the main influences on the eventual USADA case against Lance Armstrong were former teammates: Stephen Swart, Frankie Andreu, Jonathan Vaughters, Christian Vande Velde, Floyd Landis, George Hincapie, Tyler Hamilton and David Zabriskie. Landis' accusations against Armstrong were made public in 2010, and the two former friends and teammates had become antagonists.[39] Alongside evidence collected by journalists, it is arguably Landis' determination to prove that his own doping was part of a team's culture led by Armstrong that was one of the key influential factors in the latter's eventual downfall.

These riders were important, not just because they had been Armstrong's close colleagues, but also because the US Federal Inquiry of 2010–2011 had focused upon the misuse of US Government funds provided to the US Postal Services Team through sponsorship. Again we see the importance of organisations outside sport for taking the lead on anti-doping efforts. The accounts provided by Floyd Landis, Tyler Hamilton and George Hincapie motivated the US's Attorney's Office to ascertain whether some of that money had been used to purchase illegal drugs which would lead to an element of criminality beyond the sports-specific doping regulations:

> The possible crimes being investigated included the defrauding of the government, drug trafficking, money laundering and conspiracy involving Armstrong and other top cyclists. In particular, the authorities were exploring whether money from the United States Postal Service, the primary team sponsor for the first four of Armstrong's Tour de France wins, was used to buy performance-enhancing drugs ... Because the doping allegations involved activities outside the United States, the investigation focused on secondary events like the source of the money on possible drug purchases and whether Armstrong and the team

> defrauded the Postal Service when they promised to adhere to antidoping rules as part of the sponsorship agreement.[40]

When this investigation was dropped, the names of the witnesses were not made public, but detailed information was passed on to USADA. George Hincapie had not come forward voluntarily, or had any substantial accusations made against him regarding doping, but did so because of a criminal investigation. Were it not for the federal inquiry his confession may never have materialised, yet as the only rider to support Armstrong in all of his seven Tour de France wins, his influence on the process was vital:

> Among the final witnesses was Hincapie, one of the most respected riders in cycling. Antidoping officials met with him in June [2010], just days before the antidoping agency notified Armstrong of his potential doping violation. When Hincapie confessed and said Armstrong had doped and encouraged it, the antidoping agency knew it had its case.[41]

Hincapie described the moment of his decision to testify on his own personal website in October 2012:

> About two years ago, I was approached by US Federal investigators, and more recently by USADA, and asked to tell of my personal experience in these matters. I would have been much more comfortable talking only about myself, but understood that I was obligated to tell the truth about everything I knew. So that is what I did.[42]

We can see the importance of these collective accounts throughout the USADA 'Reasoned Decision', for example when their affidavits are used to support such statements as,

> In 1998 Jonny Weltz was the team director and Pedro Celaya the principal team doctor for the U.S. Postal Service Cycling Team. Riders on the team were using performance enhancing substances including EPO, testosterone, human growth hormone and cortisone.[43]

Hincapie's information provided substantial evidence, such as that he was 'generally aware that Lance was using testosterone throughout the time [Armstrong and Hincapie] were teammates'.[44] As such the build-up of information from inside US Postal was too much for Armstrong to continue his denial. Clearly, the confessions of individual cyclists were highly influential. However, these need to be set in context of the developing resources and power of anti-doping more generally.

The Power Shift towards Anti-Doping: Policy, Legal and Scientific Advances

Aside from the internal dynamics of cycling's sub-culture, which seem to have evolved (even if reluctantly) from the days of the *omerta*, the external pressures from the international anti-doping movement came to influence both at a broad organisation level and at specific moments concerning individuals.

Anti-doping policy for sport generally was a fragmented, disorganised state of affairs through the 1980s and 1990s.[45] There was very little out-of-competition testing, and anti-doping was broadly led by the International Olympic Committee who focused on their own sports and events, paying little attention to professionalised, commercialised sports like cycling, soccer, baseball and US football. The commitment to anti-doping varied between countries, some having proactive policies with Government support, others taking a *laissez-faire* approach, and others such as East Germany[46] having a policy which integrated steroid use into elite sports development systems. After the revelations from the former East Germany, the Festina scandal, speculation about Chinese athletes and ongoing evidence of doping in a number of sports, the First World Conference on Doping in Sport held in February 1999 led to the establishment of the WADA in November of that year.

It was in 1999 that Armstrong won the first of his seven consecutive Tour de France titles. That year he provided urine samples that, once a test for EPO had been established, were re-tested in 2004 and found to contain traces of the banned substance.[47] However, the lack of good scientific techniques was not the only problem facing the fledging organisation. It took five years to develop and circulate the first version of the WADA Code in 2004, which provided a definitive List of Banned Substances and standardised the two-year ban for any infringement of the Code. With the support of UNESCO, WADA lobbied all countries and all sports to become signatories to the Code. This international co-ordination was supported by an out-of-competition testing system known as 'whereabouts' in which athletes selected for a Registered Testing Pool had to provide details of their location for one hour every day to be available for testers. Moreover, the legal position of 'strict liability' underpinned the Code, meaning that the athlete is deemed responsible for any substance found in their body. Taken together, these measures strengthened the power and influence of anti-doping organisations.

While these structural-level policy initiatives set a framework for enhancing the work of anti-doping agencies, and put pressure on cycling authorities to clean up the sport, there were a number of pivotal moments. Apart from Landis and others, the eventual confession from Tyler Hamilton was central to the case against Lance Armstrong, not least because of the international media coverage generated by his appearance on the mainstream current affairs programme in the USA, *60 Minutes*.[48] Hamilton's evidence in that interview, in his award-winning autobiography, in the federal investigation and subsequent USADA investigation of the US Postal Team was instrumental in building the case against Armstrong. Indeed, it could be reasonably speculated that without Hamilton's testimony, the federal inquiry may not have been undertaken and USADA's Reasoned Decision document would not be so persuasive. However, the circumstances under which that confession eventually emerged are important ingredients in explaining the development of USADA's case and the consequences for Armstrong. Indeed, the USADA CEO Travis Tygart said that: 'It was in 2010 when Landis and Hamilton started to collaborate that we decided to start the procedure'.[49]

Hamilton's initial ban for blood doping was something of a borderline case and his appeal might have been more successful in earlier time periods when the legal apparatus underpinning anti-doping was not so uncompromising and the science of testing not as successful. A group of scientists had been working on a method for detecting blood doping, and had published their research leading to the implementation of the test at the 2004 Olympic Games. Hamilton won gold in the men's individual time trial. His 'A' sample showed a mix of blood cells that would suggest that a transfusion had been made. However, the laboratory had frozen his 'B' sample so it could not be tested. The BBC reported the incident with scepticism: 'Prosecutors want to determine if the freezing was deliberate or negligent'.[50] Indeed the Chair of the IOC Medical Commission Professor Arne Ljungqvist reported this to have been a mistake caused by heavy workload at the laboratory.[51] However, in September of the same year, Hamilton tested positive again for the same offence, this time after winning a stage of the *Vuelta a España*. Both samples were tested and USADA sanctioned Hamilton in April 2005 with a two-year ban. He appealed and the case was heard by CAS in February 2006.[52] Among a number of lines of defence, Hamilton's lawyers argued that the blood test for homologous transfusion was not sufficiently validated and that the laboratory which carried out the test had not been accredited to do so. CAS ruled that these were not grounds for an appeal and upheld the two-year ban.[53]

Hamilton's evidence was vital in building a case and gaining public interest in the matter, especially his decision to be interviewed on CBS's *60 Minutes* and to write an autobiography. Floyd Landis was another important character and, like Hamilton, the positive test that led to his confession and witness statements seems like a lucky catch for USADA and WADA. He won the 2006 Tour de France and then subsequently tested positive for testosterone. Landis was motivated to accuse Armstrong before the USADA investigation. Landis met with the Director of the Tour of California, Andrew Messick, in April 2010: 'the lunch conversation between Landis and Messick would eventually be seen as the first significant crack in Armstrong's gilded foundation, a critical turning point in antidoping officials' quest to penetrate the code of secrecy that endured in cycling'.[54] Landis had fought his ban, even going to CAS and making regular denials in public. While it transpired later he was a consistent doper, his use of testosterone during the Tour in 2006 has not been fully explained. As with Hamilton's situation, the power of anti-doping authorities, in this case the use of 'strict liability', was evidently having an effect on sport as whole. While it seemed harder to explain why testosterone would be in his system, the burden of responsibility to explain the presence of a banned substance lies with the athlete. Having failed to absolve himself, Landis wrote an autobiography and met with Messick to explain that he was not alone. The chain of events after that lunch in California is important:

> Landis's doping confession and claim that Armstrong and other Postal Service riders were involved in team-organized doping became public in May 2010, at the Tour of California. A federal investigation into Armstrong regarding doping-related crimes, including fraud and drug trafficking, ensued. The morning after the race ended, David Zabriskie – a five-time national time-trial champion and one of Armstrong's former teammates – showed up on the doorstep of the federal courthouse in Los Angeles, finally ready to tell his story.[55]

The confessions of specific cyclists cannot be clearly separated from the organisational processes that strengthened anti-doping: this is a story of intertwined, interdependent developments occurring at the levels of individual, group, sport and global policies. However, it is clear that some key witnesses only came forward because they had nowhere to turn after a positive test. In earlier times, they may have been treated more leniently. Without scientific research into new tests, a more rigorous testing system and the strict liability protocol, they may not have been sanctioned. Cyclists who came forward to help 'clean up' cycling were in fact feeling the influence of the empowerment of anti-doping – a process that began after the Festina scandal, and which has been bolstered by global legal and political structures that have led to increasing surveillance, information gathering, research on new products and techniques, and more consistent sanctioning.

Why Focus on Lance?

The analysis provided so far has offered some explanation of how anti-doping authorities increased their power and influence over cycling, and why some cyclists responded to anti-doping pressures. There were some turning points: structural changes such as the internationalisation and harmonisation of policy through WADA; high profile cyclists who came forward with details of how doping was planned, managed and anti-doping tests circumvented. Yet, even a synthesis of these themes does not fully account for the determination to catch Lance Armstrong.

The earliest accusations were made during the period 1999–2005 when he was the world's leading cyclist. The *Sunday Times* and *L'Équipe*[56] reported in 2004 on the re-testing of six samples from 1999 for EPO. However, at that time Armstrong was so confident in his position that he successfully sued the *Sunday Times* for libel. The motivation behind these media accusations based on such limited evidence that a court of law decided in favour of the cyclist is intriguing. Later accounts by the *Sunday Times* writer David Walsh suggest that there were so many rumours about Armstrong, and about the lack of post-Festina 'clean-up', that a small group of journalists decided to support anti-doping by publicising doping practices.[57] Armstrong was at the pinnacle of a doping culture and therefore would be the biggest story. Moreover, stories about less successful cyclists' doping were not gaining the public's attention. Ironically, by publishing a high profile autobiography documenting his return from cancer, by establishing the Armstrong Foundation and by creating interest in cycling through his success, Armstrong made the sport a story and made himself a story.

The first book to publicise Armstrong's doping was authored by Pierre Ballester and David Walsh. *LA Confidentiel: Les secrets des Lance Armstrong* (2004) was only published in French. It included evidence from Emma Reilly who had been Armstrong masseuse. In a move that undermined his popularity, the accused responded with a series of personal insults towards both Reilly and Walsh. Of course, Walsh was not the only writer or observer to suggest that leading cyclists were doping but he was one of the pioneers in tracking Armstrong's relationship with 'doping doctors' and interviewing those who suspected him of doping. However, when Armstrong first retired in 2005 there was no substantive evidence he had doped, his titles were his and it seems unlikely he would have been pursued with such vigour by anti-doping crusaders had he not returned to the sport in 2009.

By that year it had become more commonplace to undertake retrospective analysis of samples and to accuse athletes some years after their apparent triumph. In other sports, athletes had been stripped of their honours, for example in the case of Marion Jones. While this is an important policy process that had been ushered in, the critical questions are which athletes to target and how far back in history can anti-doping rules be applied? It is curious that the IOC has consistently refused to reassign Olympic medals despite later evidence of doping, especially in the case of East Germans.[58] The reason for targeting Armstrong seems to be that he was the most successful cyclist of the period. Yet, that seems an arbitrary and unfair criterion: why not pursue accusations against cyclists who came 2nd, 9th or 15th in Grand Tours? We could develop that further and argue that anti-doping investigations should really be universal rather than individual – all cyclists should be treated with the same energetic focus, not just the one that is successful, unpopular and making a return to the sport. Researcher Kathryn Henne recently claimed there was a certain disproportionate focus on Armstrong:

> Having ethnographically studied the anti-doping regime since 2007, I can attest that nearly every anti-doping official I have met has gone on record saying that 'catching' Armstrong would be the anti-doping movement's crowning achievement.[59]

That is not the only way in which Armstrong has been treated differently. In all other cases where a doping accusation is upheld, there is some substantial evidence. The most common form of evidence is a positive test which is confirmed by testing a 'B' sample, and which is scientifically validated by an accredited laboratory. As noted already, there is now scope to retrospectively test samples as far back as eight years. A second type of evidence is a confession, which is most common in situations where a police investigation is being conducted. If an athlete is asked by a journalist or a sports authority if they doped, they can deny without any punishments. However, if they deny in a police investigation and are later found guilty they can be prosecuted for perjury, as happened with Marion Jones. The Scottish cyclist David Millar denied doping under interrogation by the French police for almost 48 hours before eventually giving in.[60] Confessions are hard to achieve and need to be produced in very specific circumstances. Until the Lance Armstrong case, no athlete was publicly accused by a sports authority unless there was either a positive test or a confession to support the accusation.

In these circumstances, USADA took a significant risk in collecting witness statements to pursue a case for which there was little legal precedence. Their officials must have done so because of a specific determination to catch Armstrong. Given the lack of 'normal' evidence, they could have left the matter alone, but instead devoted significant resources and took significant policy risks in order to achieve their goal. However, they would not have had the details and the confidence had not the US Federal Inquiry into the financing of the US Postal Team's doping culture not begun and subsequently collapsed. The Inquiry had the power to subpoena individual cyclists, and after evidence was collected from several team members, the suspicions surrounding Armstrong were becoming public. The momentum was gathering but the Inquiry came to a halt because there was insufficient evidence to pursue a criminal case. At this stage, there was not enough supporting evidence: no positive test, no confession and no possibility of a criminal court case, USADA and WADA could have abandoned the accusation on the basis of lack of evidence, but instead the focused determination to catch Armstrong inspired more investigative work. As mentioned above, Kathryn Henne found that anti-doping staff working on professional cycling had consistently expressed a desire to catch Armstrong. Journalists felt frustrated that the fragments of evidence did not amount to a convincing case against him. However, armed with the Federal Inquiry's evidence, USADA decided to keep pursuing Armstrong. It seems that their CEO Travis Tygart was not willing to let the seven-time Tour de France winner off the hook. It is not clear if this was a personal vendetta or witch-hunt as Armstrong claimed, but certainly it seems a dogged pursuit which did not have to be undertaken. However, we should not be tempted to look solely at individuals (such as Tygart and Walsh) when in fact the wider development processes that enabled anti-doping policy were central to the unfolding outcomes of this affair.

There may have been some other influencing factors that pressurised USADA. One was that Armstrong was competing in other sports – mountain biking, triathlon and marathons – where the competitors and spectators did not tolerate suspicions of doping that had been tolerated in professional cycling. Perhaps by venturing into other areas, Armstrong unwittingly helped those who wanted to see him removed from all sports. If he had not returned in 2005 to a cleaner cycling culture and not competed in cleaner sports, he might have simply been seen as the best cyclist of a certain time period when most top cyclists were dopers and he was never caught so no accusations could stick. Instead, his desire to prove himself as an athlete in the broadest sense contributed to his eventual downfall. The fact he made enemies of important people and that USADA was determined to prove its capabilities, and that doping increasingly became a public interest story, were the other factors involved. We now know that he was doping through most of his career, but history would have told a different story had not these specific factors that – in combination with the macro- and micro-level developments already discussed – tightened the net around Armstrong.

Future: Clean Teams and Legal Nightmares?

Another factor in Armstrong's demise was the anti-doping ethos developing in a number of professional teams. This not only served to promote the values of anti-doping within cycling but also suggested to the outside world that banned substances and techniques were not necessary to be successful in cycling. One such example is Team Sky whose road race squad was built on the back of sustained achievements in track cycling. Led by David Brailsford, a rule was established that any rider with any form of doping sanction would not be invited to join Team Sky. Such was Brailsford's determination to keep up this image of a drug-free team that he refused to invite David Millar to join and Millar was allowed to join Team GB for the London 2012 Olympics (and captain the Scottish cycling team at the 2010 Commonwealth Games). Brailsford may be a pure anti-doper but the line between public and private financing is slightly blurred with Team Sky and Team GB. Government-managed National Lottery funds have supported British cycling for the Olympics and other international events. As such, any hint of doping would be highly controversial given the implied responsibility to the British public regarding the spending of Lottery funds. Another caveat to Team Sky's anti-doping regime is that the riders have benefited from a highly rationalised, scientific approach in which they are micro-managed, advised by experts, placed in a highly competitive environment and supported by new research on technology, training and nutrition. In other words, they have many forms of legal performance enhancement.

The achievements of Team Sky are quite remarkable. When Bradley Wiggins won the 2012 Tour de France, he became the first British cyclist to do so. Perhaps even more noteworthy, his early career was as a specialist short-distance track rider, quite different to the variety and distances involved in a Grand Tour. Assuming that he is not doping, the support provided by Team Sky is so extensive that he has made the change successfully from one discipline to another. During the same Tour, Wiggin's teammate Chris Froome made public his resentments that Wiggins was team leader, and claimed that he could win the Tour if given the freedom to compete against Wiggins rather than play the supportive role. He went on to achieve this in 2013, perhaps showing stronger cycling than Wiggins had in 2012 due to the lack of support from other team members (Wiggins had withdrawn before that start of the race and Geraint Thomas cracked his pelvic bone in an accident during the race). Team Sky therefore has produced two of the best cyclists in the world without resorting to doping.

We shall not know for certain if Team Sky are completely 'clean' (though there is no evidence to suggest they are cheating). History suggests that any period in which cycling authorities claim to be cracking down on doping is later found to be questionable in that respect. It is an illusion that enhanced anti-doping efforts necessarily lead to a reduction in doping. Such suspicion is not merely idle speculation. WADA and the UCI have agreed that samples can be retrospectively tested after eight years. This means that they do not believe that current athletes who do not test positive are clean: the Lance Armstrong case reinforced this perspective. It can be argued that such a policy undermines the integrity of victories, and leaves supporters unsure if the heroics of a champion are what they seem to be, as the authorities have up to eight years to overturn any result.

Even if we are now in the era of clean cycling, the USADA report into US Postal and the explicit focus on Lance Armstrong lays the foundation for some controversial future legal difficulties. One question is whether the processes used to collect evidence are to be repeated when another athlete is rumoured to have been doping, or indeed have been suspiciously too successful. A second question is how long after the doping incidents can an investigation take place. Third, how much early evidence is required to proceed with a case that involved an expensive process of tracking down and interviewing teammates, coaches, doctors and rivals? A fourth dilemma would be how many witnesses are required to make an accusation strong enough to enforce a sanction?

There are important issues for the collecting of evidence and the progressing of punishments. If this were a criminal case, the next stage would be to present the evidence in a courtroom, have witnesses cross-examined by the defence, have a judge to ensure fairness and consistency, and have a jury of peers to decide the outcome. At present, the accused is given the opportunity of arbitration after the evidence has been made public and decisions are made by a panel of three adjudicators. This would take place in CAS, which is designed to uphold the principles of sport. If a doping charge went to a criminal court and the jury were not sports fans or experts, and decisions made without recourse to socially constructed notions of 'value' in sports, then it might be found that the non-risky, consenting use of drugs when most others are doing so is not really a crime. Even in the East German court cases, the only 'crime' that the doping leaders were convicted of was 'abuse of minors'. The distribution of steroids to adults was not considered serious enough to be penalised by the criminal justice process. In the grander scheme of things, the worst accusation that can be made against Armstrong and others who have doped is that they have contravened an apparently sacred notion of 'fairness'. This is hardly a crime to warrant the time and resources of criminal investigators or state legal processes. 'Fairness' in sport is an arbitrary concept, applied more rigorously to drug-taking than to other incidents like shirt-pulling in soccer, stamping in rugby or punching below the belt in boxing. Moreover, little or no physical harm has come to any of the US Postal Team, and they were consenting adults who knew the risks (even if influenced by key figures and the sport's doping culture). 'Health' is another arbitrary concept: why are cyclists encouraged to fly down mountains and take hair-pin bends as fast as possible but are not allowed to take medically tested and supervised drugs to combat fatigue?

This leads to a final comment about the principles of anti-doping. The regulatory document – the WADA Code – states that the purpose of the Code and the worldwide anti-doping programme is: 'To protect the Athletes' fundamental right to participate in doping-free sport and thus promote health, fairness and equality for Athletes worldwide'.[61] It could be argued in defence of Lance Armstrong and cyclists of the 'doping era' that: (1) their rights to participate in doping-free sport were not respected and protected; (2) their health was not damaged by doping; (3) even if it was, it was their own choice; and (4) the 'omerta' served to give cyclists the equality of doping. The intrusion of anti-doping has created chaos, new forms of unfairness, ruined lives and reputations, and potentially created problematic consequences for future sports. The wider context of the Lance Armstrong case is about more than one person; it is about processes and decisions with intriguing motives and uncertain outcomes.

Acknowledgements

The author would like to thank the Fulbright Commission, Thomas M. Hunt and the staff and students of the H.J. Lutcher Stark Center, University of Texas, and Verner Møller.

Notes on Contributor

Paul Dimeo is a Senior Lecturer at the University of Stirling. He has researched various aspects of drug use in sport and anti-doping policies.

Notes

1. USADA, *Report on Proceedings*.
2. *Telegraph*, "Lance Armstrong Oprah Winfrey."
3. See, for example, Walsh, *Seven Deadly Sins*; Strickland, "Lance Armstrong's End Game"; and McCann, "Armstrong's Confession."
4. Halliburton, "Armstrong Asks Judge."

5. For an insightful discussion of the ethics of stripping Armstrong of his titles, see Gleaves, "Saying It's So."
6. There is an extensive literature on the historical and contemporary relationship of cycling and doping which cannot be fully utilised given the scope of this article. Aside from the texts cited here, readers might find the following valuable and interesting: Dimeo, *A History of Drug*; Møller, *The Doping Devil*; Whittle, *Bad Blood*; and López, "Creating Fear."
7. The German Tour de France 1997 winner Jan Ullrich admitted doping during his career in June 2013, and claimed: 'For me, betrayal only begins when I gain an advantage, but that was not the case. I just wanted to ensure equal opportunities' (BBC, "Jan Ullrich").
8. Hoberman, "Sports Physicians"; Hoberman, "A Pharmacy on Wheels"; Waddington, *Sport, Health and Drugs*; Walsh, *Seven Deadly Sins*; and Donati, "Anti-Doping."
9. Møller, *The Ethics of Doping*.
10. Walsh, *Seven Deadly Sins*.
11. Voet, *Breaking the Chain*.
12. These quotes from Obree were provided originally to the *Independent* and *L'Equipe*, and are cited on Wikipedia, "Graeme Obree." His achievements in other cycle events demonstrate that he had the potential to develop a successful professional career were it not for the perceived necessity of doping.
13. Cited in Waddington, *Sport, Health and Drugs*, 180.
14. Hamilton and Coyle, *The Secret Race*.
15. Brewer, "Commercialization in Professional Cycling"; Woodland, *The Crooked Path*; and Hoberman, "A Pharmacy on Wheels."
16. Møller, *The Ethics of Doping*, 49.
17. Waddington, *Sport, Health and Drugs*, 166.
18. USADA, *Report on Proceedings*, 22.
19. Hoberman, "A Pharmacy on Wheels," 108.
20. Hoberman, "A Pharmacy on Wheels," 107.
21. Møller, *The Ethics of Doping*, 19.
22. Millar, *Racing Through the Dark*.
23. USADA, *Report on Proceedings*, 24.
24. Kimmage, "Cycling."
25. Walsh, *From Lance to Landis*, cited in Kimmage, "Cycling."
26. USADA, *Report on Proceedings*, 172.
27. Møller, *The Ethics of Doping*, 58. Møller here refers to 'sport' more widely. The focus of this article remains on cycling, but it is important to note that other sports have a historical record of doping incidents. Cycling has been the focus of much anti-doping effort, and in a sense this is self-producing. More tests mean more positives; while other sports appear to be 'cleaner', it may simply be that fewer tests are being carried out.
28. Christiansen, "The Legacy of Festina."
29. Donegan, "Has Everybody Stopped Caring."
30. Walsh, *Seven Deadly Sins*.
31. Kimmage, *Rough Ride*, 229.
32. Voet, *Breaking the Chain*, 127–8.
33. BBC, "Peddlers."
34. Christiansen, "The Legacy of Festina," 151.
35. Ibid.
36. DeCanio, "The Stolen Underground Story."
37. Cycling News, "Millar Confesses."
38. Wikipedia, "Michael Rasmussen"; for a critical account of these decisions, see Møller, *The Scapegoat*.
39. *USA Today*, "Lance Armstrong Makes Public."
40. Austen, "Inquiry on Lance Armstrong."
41. Macur, "Armstrong's Wall of Silence."
42. Hincapie, "Statement from George Hincapie."
43. USADA, *Report on Proceedings*, 16.
44. Ibid., 39.
45. Houlihan, *Dying to Win*; Hunt, Dimeo and Jedlicka, "Anti-doping Policy."
46. Dimeo, Hunt and Horbury, "The Individual"; Dennis and Grix, *Sport under Communism*.

47. Ruibal, "Armstrong Had Six Positives."
48. For details, see Bicycling, "The Full Tyler Hamilton."
49. Tour de José, "Translation of Travis."
50. BBC, "Hamilton Faces Greek Drug Probe."
51. *VeloNews*, "Olympic Case Dropped Against Tyler Hamilton."
52. CAS, *Arbitral Award.*
53. Ibid.
54. Macur, "Armstrong's Wall of Silence."
55. Ibid.
56. *L'Équipe*, September 26, 2012.
57. Walsh, *Seven Deadly Sins.*
58. Hersch, "If Armstrong Loses Olympic Medal."
59. Henne, "Doped or Duped?"
60. Millar, *Racing Through the Dark.*
61. WADA, *World Anti-Doping Code*, 11.

References

Austen, I. "Inquiry on Lance Armstrong Ends With No Charges." *International Herald Tribune*, February 3. Accessed February 10. http://www.nytimes.com/2012/02/04/sports/cycling/federal-prosecutors-drop-lance-armstrong-investigation.html?_r=0, 2012.

BBC. "Hamilton Faces Greek Drug Probe." December 20. Accessed January 16, 2013. http://news.bbc.co.uk/sport1/hi/other_sports/cycling/4111071.stm, 2004.

BBC. "Jan Ullrich: Former Tour de France Winner Admits Blood Doping." June 22, 2013. Accessed June 28, 2013. http://www.bbc.co.uk/sport/0/cycling/23013133, 2013.

BBC. "Peddlers – Cycling's Dirty Truth." Radio 5, October 15 2012.

Bicycling. "The Full Tyler Hamilton Interview: The Price of Truth." December 19. Accessed July 23, 2013. http://www.bicycling.co.za/news-people/people/the-full-tyler-hamilton-interview-the-price-of-truth/, 2012.

Brewer, B. "Commercialization in Professional Cycling, 1950–2001: Institutional Transformation and the Rationalization of 'Doping'." *Sociology of Sport* 19 (2002): 276–301.

Christiansen, A. V. "The Legacy of Festina: Patterns of Drug Use in European Cycling Since 1998." In *Drugs, Alcohol and Sport*, edited by P. Dimeo, 144–161. London: Routledge, 2007.

Court of Arbitration for Sport [CAS]. *Arbitral Award, CAS 2005/A/884 Tyler Hamilton v USADA/UCI*, 2006.

Cycling News. "Millar Confesses." June 25. Accessed January 30, 2013. http://autobus.cyclingnews.com/news.php?id=news/2004/jun04/jun25news3, 2004.

DeCanio, M. "The Stolen Underground Story." Accessed February 15, 2013. http://www.stolenunderground.com/matt_decanio_s_story__join_social_network_

Dennis, M., and J. Grix. *Sport under Communism: Behind the East German "Miracle"*. Palgrave Macmillan: Basingstoke, 2012.

Dimeo, P. *A History of Drug Use in Sport, 1876–1976: Beyond Good and Evil*. London: Routledge, 2007.

Dimeo, P., T. Hunt, and R. Horbury. "The Individual and the State: A Social Historical Analysis of the East German Doping System." *Sport in History* 31, no. 3 (2011): 218–237.

Donati, S. "Anti-Doping: The Fraud Behind the Stage." Paper presented at the Play the Game conference. Accessed June 24, 2013. http://www.vivamarathon.dk/anti_dopin.pdf, 2006.

Donegan, L. "Has Everybody Stopped Caring About Doping in Sport?" *Guardian*, August 6, 2009. Accessed February 8, 2013. http://www.guardian.co.uk/sport/blog/2009/aug/06/drugs-doping-boston-red-sox-bath-rugby, 2009.

Gleaves, J. "Saying It's So: Lance Armstrong and Doping." Commentary for the International Network of Humanistic Doping Research. Accessed January 21, 2013. http://ph.au.dk/en/about-the-department-of-public-health/sections/sektion-for-idraet/forskning/forskningsenheden-sport-og-kropskultur/international-network-of-humanistic-doping-research/online-resources/commentaries/saying-its-so-lance-armstrong-and-doping/, 2012.

Halliburton, S. "Armstrong Asks Judge to Dismiss a $12 Million Suit." *Austin Statesman*, April 6. Accessed June 27, 2013. http://www.statesman.com/news/sports/armstrong-asks-judge-to-dismiss-a-12-million-suit-/nXFQc/, 2013.

Hamilton, T., and D. Coyle. *The Secret Race: Inside the Hidden World of the Tour de France: Doping, Cover-ups, and Winning at All Costs*. London: Transworld, 2012.
Henne, K. "Doped or Duped? Legacies of Anti-Doping Regulation in the Wake of Lance Armstrong." Commentary for the International Network of Humanistic Doping Research. Accessed January 20, 2013. http://ph.au.dk/en/about-the-department-of-public-health/sections/sektion-for-idraet/forskning/forskningsenheden-sport-og-kropskultur/international-network-of-humanistic-doping-research/online-resources/commentaries/doped-or-duped-legacies-of-anti-doping-regulation-in-the-wake-of-lance-armstrong/, 2012.
Hersch, P. "If Armstrong Loses Olympic Medal, Why Not East Germans?" *Chicago Herald Tribune*, December 11. Accessed July 13, 2013. http://articles.chicagotribune.com/2012-12-11/sports/chi-if-armstrong-loses-olympic-medal-why-not-east-germans-20121211_1_uci-usada-ioc-executive-board, 2012.
Hincapie, G. "Statement from George Hincapie." October 10. Accessed February 8, 2013. http://www.georgehincapie.com/news/Statement-from-George-Hincapie/, 2012.
Hoberman, J. "'A Pharmacy on Wheels': Doping and Community Cohesion among Professional Cyclists Following the Tour de France Scandal of 1998." In *The Essence of Sport*, edited by V. Møller, and J. Nauright, 107–127. Odense: University of Southern Denmark Press, 2003.
Hoberman, J. "Sports Physicians and the Doping Crisis in Elite Sport." *Clinical Journal of Sport Medicine* 12, no. 4 (2002): 203–208.
Houlihan, B. *Dying to Win: Doping in Sport and the Development of Anti-Doping Policy*. Strasbourg: Council of Europe, 1999.
Hunt, T., P. Dimeo, and S. Jedlicka. "Anti-Doping Policy, 1960–2000: A Critical Historical Perspective on Contemporary Problems." *Performance Enhancement and Health* 1, no. 2 (2012): 55–60.
Kimmage, P. "Cycling: Big Reveal of Cancer Jesus." *Independent*, October 21. Accessed January 10, 2013. http://www.independent.ie/sport/other-sports/cycling-big-reveal-of-cancer-jesus-3266380.html, 2012.
Kimmage, P. *Rough Ride*. London: Yellow Jersey, 1998.
L'Équipe. (September 26, 2012), cited by website Stolen Underground Run by Matt DeCanio. Accessed January 16, 2013. http://su13.us/news?blogstart=39
López, B. "Creating Fear: The 'Doping Deaths', Risk Communication and the Anti-Doping Campaign." *International Journal of Sports Policy and Politics*, published online 2013. doi:10.1080/19406940.2013.773359.
Macur, J. "Armstrong's Wall of Silence Fell Rider by Rider." *New York Times*, October 20. Accessed February 12. http://www.nytimes.com/2012/10/21/sports/how-armstrongs-wall-fell-one-rider-at-a-time.html?pagewanted=all&_r=1&, 2012.
McCann, M. "Armstrong's Confession to Have Stark, Wide-Reaching Impact." *Sports Illustrated*, January 18. Accessed June 26, 2013. http://sportsillustrated.cnn.com/more/news/20130118/lance-armstrong-legal-implications/, 2013.
Millar, D. *Racing Through the Dark: The Fall and Rise of David Millar*. London: Orion, 2011.
Møller, V. *The Doping Devil*. Norderstedt: Books on Demand, 1999[2008].
Møller, V. *The Ethics of Doping and Anti-Doping: Redeeming the Soul of Sport?* London: Routledge, 2010.
Møller, V. *The Scapegoat, About the Expulsion of Michael Rasmussen from the Tour De France 2007 and Beyond*. Aarhus: Akaprint, 2011.
Ruibal, S. "Armstrong Had Six Positives from 1999 Tests." USA Today. Accessed January 10, 2013. http://usatoday30.usatoday.com/sports/cycling/2005-08-24-armstrong-samples-details_x.htm 2004.
Strickland, B. "Lance Armstrong's End Game." *Bicycling Magazine*, March 2013. Accessed June 25, 2013. http://www.bicycling.com/news/pro-cycling/lance-armstrongs-endgame 2013.
Telegraph. "Lance Armstrong Oprah Winfrey Interview Watched by 28 Million." January 23. Accessed January 29, 2013. http://www.telegraph.co.uk/sport/othersports/cycling/lancearmstrong/9820162/Lance-Armstrong-Oprah-Winfrey-interview-watched-by-28-million.html 2013.
Tour de José. "Translation of Travis Tygart's Interview with *L'Équipe*." September 24. Accessed July 11, 2013. http://tourdejose.com/2012/09/24/transcript-of-travis-tygarts-interview-with-lequipe/, 2012.
United States Anti-Doping Agency (USADA). *Report on Proceedings under the World Anti-Doping Code and the USADA Protocol; United States Anti-Doping Agency, Claimant v. Lance*

Armstrong, Respondent; Reasoned Decision of the United States Anti-Doping Agency on Disqualification and Ineligibility. Colorado Springs: USADA, 2012.
USA Today. "Lance Armstrong Makes Public Emails from Floyd Landis." May 22. Accessed July 24, 2013. http://usatoday30.usatoday.com/sports/cycling/2010-05-21-armstrong-landis-emails_N.htm, 2010.
VeloNews. "Olympic Case Dropped Against Tyler Hamilton: Still Facing Vuelta Sanctions." September 23. http://www.freerepublic.com/focus/f-news/1226633/posts, 2004.
Voet, W., translated by William Fotheringham *Breaking the Chain: Drugs and Cycling – The True Story*. London: Yellow Jersey, 2001.
WADA. *World Anti-Doping Code*. Montreal: WADA, 2009.
Waddington, I. *Sport, Health and Drugs: A Critical Sociological Perspective*. London: Spon, 2000.
Walsh, D. *From Lance to Landis: Inside the American Doping Controversy at the Tour de France*. New York: Ballantine, 2007.
Walsh, D. *Seven Deadly Sins – My Pursuit of Lance Armstrong*. London: Simon & Schuster, 2012.
Whittle, J. *Bad Blood: The Secret Life of the Tour de France*. London: Yellow Jersey, 2009.
Wikipedia. "Graeme Obree." Accessed July 24, 2013. http://en.wikipedia.org/wiki/Graeme_Obree
Wikipedia. "Michael Rasmussen." Accessed July 18, 2013. http://en.wikipedia.org/wiki/Michael_Rasmussen
Woodland, L. *The Crooked Path to Victory: Drugs and Cheating in Professional Bicycle Racing*. San Francisco, CA: Cycle, 2003.

Index

Note: Page numbers followed by 'n' refer to notes